GENIUS AND PARTNERSHIP: ANCEL AND MARGARET KEYS AND THE DISCOVERY OF THE MEDITERRANEAN DIET

GENIUS AND PARTNERSHIP: ANCEL AND MARGARET KEYS AND THE DISCOVERY OF THE MEDITERRANEAN DIET

JOSEPH L. DIXON

Joseph L. Dixon Publishing
New Brunswick, NJ

Book Cover Design: Peter Serko. Bottle of aged balsamic vinegar was from the Glover Street Market, Twisp, WA, 98856.

Credits for Collage of Cook Book Covers in Chapter 8:

Jacket Design from EAT WELL AND STAY WELL by Ancel and Margaret Keys. Jacket Design Copyright © 1959 by William Meek. Reprinted with the acknowledgment of Penguin Random House LLC (which Doubleday & Company, Inc. is now part of).

Jacket Design from THE BENEVOLENT BEAN by Margaret and Ancel Keys. Jacket Design Copyright © 1967 by Ruth Deardoff. Reprinted by permission of Farrar, Straus and Giroux, LLC.

Jacket Design from HOW TO EAT WELL AND STAY WELL THE MEDITERRANEAN WAY by Ancel and Margaret Keys. Jacket Illustration Copyright © 1975 by Ron Becker. Jacket Typography Copyright © 1975 by Lewis Friedman. Reprinted with the acknowledgment of Penguin Random House LLC (which Doubleday & Company, Inc. is now part of).

First Edition, March 2015

Interior designed by JL Dixon using Pressbooks.com (Asimov theme)

ISBN:

978-0-9862955-0-8 (Ebook Version)

978-0-9862955-1-5 (Softcover Version)

978-0-9862955-2-2 (Hard Cover Version)

For Patrick, Angelina, and Marisa

CONTENTS

Why I Wrote about Ancel Keys xi

Time Line for the Life of Ancel Keys xiv

Updates, Footnotes, Hyperlinks, Figures, Index, Cover Design, and Credits xx

PART I. ANCEL KEYS AND THE SEVEN COUNTRIES STUDY

1. The Visionary Who Started It All 3
2. How the Seven Countries Study was Conceived 10
3. Implementing the Seven Countries Study 19
4. A Closer Look at Seven Countries 30
5. The "Something Else Hypothesis" - A Insidious Cause of Increased Coronary Heart Disease in the U.S. in the 1950s 49
6. The Keyses in the Lab; Contribution to the Discovery of LDL 62
7. The Fat and Cholesterol Human Feeding Studies of the 1950s and 1960s 71

8. After Seven Countries-Retirement, Life in Italy, and Scientific Legacy 79

9. A Successful Collaboration Continues the Seven Countries Study 93

PART II. CHOLESTEROL: WHAT IS IT?

10. Drs. Goldstein and Brown Discover the LDL Receptor 109

11. Why is There Cholesterol in the Body? 120

12. The Framingham Study, the Mount Everest of Epidemiological Studies 137

13. Discovery of the Statin Drugs, Rollback of LDL, and Protection from CHD 153

14. Even When Your Cholesterol Levels Are Perfect, Avoid That Second Slice of Cheesecake 163

PART III. LIVING THE MEDITERRANEAN WAY

15. Living the Mediterranean Way: Discovery of the Mediterranean Diet 179

16. What We Know About the Mediterranean Diet Today 192

17. Genius and Partnership 202

Appendix 217

Glossary 221

Acknowledgments 230

About the Author 232

WHY I WROTE ABOUT ANCEL KEYS

I wrote this book on Ancel Keys and the origin of the cholesterol hypothesis for several reasons.

First, I have been teaching a course called "Nutrition and Health" for almost 25 years and I have taught the material in this book many times. Over this period of time I have adjusted my teaching so that my students could maximally learn the important concepts underlying cholesterol and lipoprotein metabolism and could draw from this information in later classes.

Second, I have been asked by many people about cholesterol and why it is so important or so bad for them. I finally decided to write a book that would finally explain the functions of this mystery substance in a way that my friends and family could understand. In fact, I have encountered some doctors who had no idea what cholesterol was and what it did in the body. So this book is for them, too.

Third, one day I started to look through Ancel Keys's *Seven Countries* book that I had on my office bookshelf. I kept on reading it through the afternoon, and by the next day, I had read the book cover to cover. And the thought that immediately came to my mind was that everything that I had heard about Ancel Keys in my graduate school classes and in basic scientific discussions was not accurate. I had heard that he had been a dominant and divisive figure in the history of coronary heart disease research, but this was not the Ancel Keys that came across so eloquently in *Seven Countries*. The book was carefully written and was open minded; Ancel Keys did not use bombastic language or imply that he was the ultimate source of knowledge; and most importantly, several times in the book he acknowledged that he did not understand particular findings. I found a man who was a true scientist, and not someone who used science for his own purposes and advancement.

Then I read the cookbook, *How to Eat Well and Stay Well the Mediterranean Way*, that Dr. Keys and Margaret Keys wrote. I couldn't believe my eyes. It was a wonderful book that reviewed how they became interested in the Mediterranean diet. And it contained many wonderful and healthy recipes, too. And as he does in his scientific research articles and his book, *Seven Countries*, Dr. Keys and Margaret give credit to other scientists who influenced their ideas.

Today if one searches for Ancel Keys on the internet, it is immediately apparent that there are many activists who consider him evil because of his scientific findings. They dispute the cholesterol hypothesis with very little understanding concerning how complex lipid metabolism is, and with little sense of how much work is required to make even elementary scientific discoveries. In fact, they remind me of the global warming science deniers that are so prevalent today. So another reason I wrote this book was to set the record straight not only concerning Ancel Keys's research accomplishments, but also the research of the many scientists who have struggled to make sense of the cholesterol and fat fields.

This book focuses on Ancel Keys and the pursuit of the early basic knowledge concerning coronary heart disease and the effects of diet on cholesterol concentrations in the blood. Except in specific cases, I have not reported on more recent studies, nor have I discussed the scientists who were involved in recent research that has expanded our information on cholesterol and lipoprotein metabolism. Two recently published books are excellent resources for information concerning research on cholesterol and coronary heart disease: Dr. Daniel Steinberg published *The Cholesterol Wars* in 2007.[1] Dr. A. Stewart Truswell published *Cholesterol and Beyond* in 2010.[2] Each of these books cite close to 1000 references that document specific observations and experiments on cholesterol and lipid nutrition and metabolism.

1. Steinberg D. (2007) *The Cholesterol Wars, The Skeptics vs. the Preponderance of Evidence.* Amsterdam: Academic Press (Elsevier).
2. Truswell AS. (2010) *Cholesterol and Beyond, The Research on Diet and Coronary Heart Disease 1900-2000.* Dordrecht: Springer Science.

TIME LINE FOR THE LIFE OF ANCEL KEYS

Time Line for Dr. Ancel Keys

1904	Ancel Keys was born in Colorado on January 26, 1904
1922	Entered University of California-Berkeley
1928	Started graduate assistantship at Scripps Institute of Oceanography, La Jolla, California
1930	Received Ph.D. from Berkeley; Traveled to Copenhagen to work with Dr. August Krogh, a Nobel Prize-winning physiologist
1931	Transferred to University of Cambridge, England, to work with Dr. Joseph Barcroft on high-altitude physiology
1933	Received Ph.D. from King's College, Cambridge University; Headed to Harvard University for a faculty position at the Harvard Fatigue Laboratory
1935	Conducted six-month expedition to Andes Mountains to perform high-altitude physiology experiments
1937	Started at Mayo Clinic, Rochester, Minnesota; Hired Ms. Margaret Haney as a laboratory technician
1938	Dr. Ancel Keys recruited by the University of Minnesota; Established Laboratory of Physiological Hygiene
1939	Ancel Keys and Margaret Haney married
1940	The Keyses' first child, Caroline, was born
1941	Dr. Keys was asked by the Army to develop a mobile, nutritious, combat ration–later called K rations
1942	The Keyses' second child, Henry, was born
1943	Dr. Keys wrote a comprehensive proposal to study starvation in 36 conscientious objector volunteers
1944	Starvation Study started with conscientious objectors at University of Minnesota
1945	Report sent to War Department on how to care for starved humans; Starvation Study ends October, 1945

1946	Published: Ancel Keys, Human Starvation and Its Consequences, *J Am Dietetic Assoc* 22:582-587, 1946
1947	Dr. Keys and Minnesota colleagues begin Minnesota Business and Professional Men Study (studied diet-coronary heart disease association)
1949	The Keyses' third child, Martha, was born
1950	*The Biology of Human Starvation* published in two volumes by the University of Minnesota Press (1,200 pages)
1951	Ancel and Margaret Keys and family traveled to Oxford, England, on Fulbright Award
1952	Ancel and Margaret Keys traveled to Naples, Italy, and Spain to confirm low rates of coronary heart disease
1953	Seminar at Mt. Sinai Hospital in New York City where Dr. Keys used Food and Agriculture Organization and World Health Organization ecological health data to propose a hypothesis concerning a diet-coronary heart disease connection
1954	Geneva meeting where Sir George Pickering of Oxford questioned and attacked Dr. Keys's diet-coronary heart disease hypothesis. A. Keys returned to Naples, Italy with Paul White; Dr. Noboru Kimura from Japan visited the United States; Dr. Blackburn joined the Laboratory of Physiological Hygiene
1955	A. and M. Keys visited Cape Town, South Africa, and published: B. Bronte-Stewart, A. Keys, J.F. Brock, with the collaboration of A.D. Moodie, M.H. Keys, A. Antonis. Serum-cholesterol, diet, and coronary heart disease, an inter-racial survey in the Cape Peninsula. *Lancet*, Nov 26 1955, 1103-1108. This is one of the first reports that diet-induced increased blood cholesterol occurs due to an increase in LDL-cholesterol; Ancel Keys visited Hawaii and Japan.
1956	Dr. Keys began a collaboration with Professor Martti Karvonen of the Institute of Occupational Health in Helsinki, Finland, and visited East Karelia. A. Keys returned to Hawaii and Japan, and visited the Soviet Union with Paul White.
1957	A. Keys visited Nicotera, Italy, and Crete and Corfu, Greece, as part of the pre-studies for the Seven Countries Study
1958	Seven Countries Study officially started in Yugoslavia, Tanushimaru in southern Japan, and in the United States as part of the U.S. Railroad Study

1959 *Eat Well and Stay Well,* published by Doubleday, and serialized in newspapers; Seven Countries Study started in East and West Finland

1960 Studies started in Ushibuka, Japan; Crevalcore and Montegiogio, Italy; Zutphen, Netherlands; and Crete, Greece

1961 Dr. Ancel Keys appeared on cover of *Time* magazine (January 13, 1961 issue); Studies started in Corfu, Greece

1962 Rome Railroad Study started; Studies started in Yelika Krsna, Serbia

1963 Ancel and Margaret Keys purchased land south of Naples and later built a home and named it "Minnelea"; Studies started in Zrenjanin, Serbia

1964 Seven Countries Studies started in Belgrade, Yugoslavia (Serbia) (Last cohort to start)

1965 Published: Series of four papers in the journal, *Metabolism*, on the dietary fat and cholesterol human feeding studies carried out in the Keys's laboratory

1967 *The Benevolent Bean*, published by Doubleday & Co.; Published monograph: Keys A. and colleagues. Epidemiological studies related to coronary heart disease. Characteristics of men aged 40-59 in Seven Countries. *Acta Med Scand* 460(Suppl.180):392 pp.

1970 Published: Keys A. (Editor). Coronary heart disease in seven countries. Multiple articles, *Circulation* 1970;41(Suppl.1):211 pp.

1972 A. Keys retired from the University of Minnesota; Dr. Henry Blackburn appointed as head of the Laboratory of Physiological Hygiene

1975 *How to Eat Well and Stay Well the Mediterranean Way*, published by Doubleday

1976 Published additional studies on cholesterol feeding in order to confirm earlier results: Anderson, Grande, and Keys. Independence of the effects of cholesterol and degree of saturation of the fat in the diet on serum cholesterol in man. *Am. J. Clin. Nutr.* 29: 1784-1789, 1976

1977	Landmark report from the Framingham Study: Gordon T. and colleagues. High density lipoprotein as a protective factor against coronary heart disease. The Framingham Study. *Am J Med.* 162(5):707-14; U.S. Congressional Select Committee (McGovern committee) issued the "Dietary Goals for the United States." There was no correspondence indicating Dr. Keys played a direct role in advising the McGovern committee
1980	*Seven Countries*, by Ancel Keys and colleagues, published by Harvard University Press
1985	Published: Keys A. and colleagues. Serum cholesterol and cancer mortality in the Seven Countries Study. *Am J Epidemiol* 121: 870-883
1986	Published: Keys A. and colleagues. The diet and 15-year death rate in the seven countries study. *Am J Epidemiol.* 124(6): 903-15
1994	Monograph published: Kromhout D, Menotti A, Blackburn H (Eds). (1994) *The Seven Countries Study: A scientific adventure in cardiovascular disease epidemiology.* Brouwer Offset b.v., Utrecht; Published: Vartiainen and colleagues, Changes in risk factors explain changes in mortality from ischaemic heart disease in Finland. *BMJ.* 1994; 309: 23–27. In 25 years, mortality from coronary heart disease in Finland decreased to less than half its original level
1995	Published: Keys A. Mediterranean diet and public health: personal reflections. *Am J Clin Nutr.* 1995 Jun;61(6 Suppl):1321S-1323S
1996	Dr. Henry Blackburn retired from the University of Minnesota, but continues to this day as advisor to the Seven Countries Study
1999	Published: Menotti A. and colleagues. Food intake patterns and 25-year mortality from coronary heart disease: Cross-cultural correlations in the Seven Countries Study. *Eur J of Epidemiol* 15: 507-515
2002	Monograph published: Kromhout D, Menotti A, Blackburn H (Eds). *Prevention of coronary heart disease. Diet, lifestyle and risk factors in the Seven Countries Study.* Kluwer Academic Publishers, Boston, 2002. 267 pp.
2004	Ancel Keys died in Minneapolis on November 20, 2004, two months short of his 101st birthday
2006	Margaret Keys died at the age of 97; Todd Tucker published: *The Great Starvation Experiment*, Free Press (Simon & Schuster), New York

2007	Published: Menotti A. and colleagues. Forty-year coronary mortality trends and changes in Seven Countries Study. *Eur J Epidemiol* 22: 747–754
2014	Alessandro Menotti, Dann Kromhout, Henry Blackburn, and David R Jacobs Jr. 50-year follow-up data of the Seven Countries Study completed and in preparation for publication

UPDATES, FOOTNOTES, HYPERLINKS, FIGURES, INDEX, COVER DESIGN, AND CREDITS

Updates–Due to the revolution in publishing that has occurred in the past few years, this is a living book that will be updated if events and findings call for it. Therefore, the E version of this book will be updated periodically. As this book goes to press (March 1, 2015) a leaked report from the U.S. Dietary Guideline Committee[1] suggests that the recommendation to limit cholesterol intake will be dropped from the upcoming U.S. Dietary Guidelines. As a historical note, the feeding studies conducted by Ancel Keys in the 1950s (See Chapter 7) definitively showed that going from an intake of essentially zero mg of cholesterol per day to about 300 to 400 mg per day in adult males raised blood cholesterol about 7-8 mg/dL. Whereas this small increase is significant when considering 100s of millions of people, there are many ways to lower blood cholesterol today. The concern is to not frighten people from consuming eggs, a very good source of protein for people–especially the

1. http://www.washingtonpost.com/blogs/wonkblog/wp/2015/02/10/feds-poised-to-withdraw-longstanding-warnings-about-dietary-cholesterol/

elderly and certain vegetarians. Of course, the recommendations on saturated fat intake remain. Saturated fat has a much greater influence on blood cholesterol concentrations. I have a feeling that Dr. Keys would support this change in the U.S. Dietary Guidelines.

Please send your notes, suggestions, and corrections to dixon@aesop.rutgers.edu

Corrections since the first Ebook and soft cover printed book were produced–On February 21, 2016, In Chapter 4, the Figure Legend to Figure 14.2 from *Seven Countries* (1980) was corrected as some of the countries were misidentified on the graph. Also, two small corrections were found by Ms. Carrie D'Andrea (Carrie Keys, daughter of Ancel and Margaret Keys) and corrected: On page 25, Dr. Victorio Pudda's name was misspelled (now Correct) and on page 43, the title of *How to Eat Well and Stay Well the Mediterranean Way* (1975) was corrected.

Footnotes–For readability, footnotes were kept to a reasonable number per chapter. For published journal articles, I have included a hyperlink to an article if it was available at the time of publication. If only an abstract was available, the hyperlink is usually to the citation in the Pubmed database (US National Library of Medicine, National Institutes of Health). There are also hyperlinks to websites that contain additional information about Dr. Keys. Of special note is the website maintained by Dr. Henry Blackburn at the University of Minnesota Division of Epidemiology and Community Health: http://www.epi.umn.edu/cvdepi

References–Two comprehensive books on cholesterol have recently been published and each contains close to 1000 citations. Additional references can be obtained from these two books.[2 3]

2. Steinberg D. (2007) *The Cholesterol Wars, The Skeptics vs. the Preponderance of Evidence.* Amsterdam: Academic Press (Elsevier).
3. Truswell AS. (2010) *Cholesterol and Beyond, The Research on Diet and Coronary Heart Disease 1900-2000.* Dordrecht: Springer Science.

Figures–Many figures were drawn by the author and can be viewed in a larger format by clicking on the figure when you are reading the pdf version on line.

Index–An index was not prepared. When reading the pdf or E versions, use the search function in order to find terms, places, and individuals. There is a short Glossary of the most commonly used terms in the back matter of the book.

Cover Design–The cover design and photograph were by Peter Serko (PeterSerko.com). The bottle on the cover is aged balsamic vinegar from the Glover Street Market, 124 N. Glover St., Twisp, WA, 98856 (gloverstreetmarket.com).

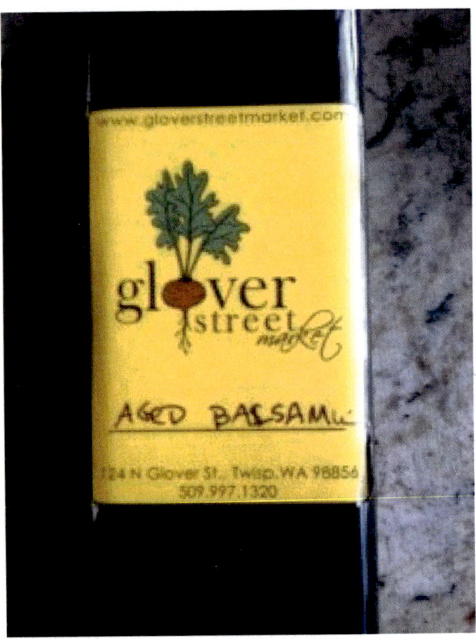

Aged balsamic vinegar from the Glover Street Market, Twisp, WA, 98856.

Credits–Permissions were obtained to use the images from other sources that appear throughout this book. In Chapter 8 the photograph of the collage of cookbook covers from the cookbooks by Ancel and Maragret Keys was by JL Dixon. The cover images were used by permission of Penguin Random House LLC (which Doubleday & Company, Inc. is now part of) and Farrar, Straus and Giroux, LLC (which published The Benevolent Bean in 1972). The designers for the original covers were as follows: Jacket Design for EAT WELL AND STAY WELL by Ancel and Margaret Keys, Copyright © 1959 by William Meek; Jacket Design for THE BENEVOLENT BEAN by Margaret and Ancel Keys, Copyright © 1967 by Ruth Deardoff. Jacket Design for HOW TO EAT WELL AND STAY WELL THE MEDITERRANEAN WAY by Ancel and Margaret Keys, Illustration Copyright © 1975 by Ron Becker, Typography Copyright © 1975 by Lewis Friedman.

In some versions of the book the cover image included columns from a photograph, "Temple_Of_Olmpian_Zeus" by AlMare. The original file is at: http://commons.wikimedia.org/wiki/File:Temple_Of_Olmpian_Zeus_retouched.jpg

The image of the columns is licensed under the Creative Commons Attribution-Share Alike 2.5 Generic license (http://creativecommons.org/licenses/by-sa/2.5/deed.en).

PART I.

ANCEL KEYS AND THE SEVEN COUNTRIES STUDY

1.

THE VISIONARY WHO STARTED IT ALL

If you Google Ancel Keys today you will see a group of websites that vilify Ancel Keys and call him the original source for the "Cholesterol Myth." The "Cholesterol Myth" is the term used for the idea that all of the research that focused on dietary saturated fat and cholesterol and blood cholesterol concentration as important causative factors for coronary heart disease was incorrect and, in fact, the whole concept was a conspiracy to make the American people eat a certain way. One question that immediately comes to mind is, if the "Cholesterol Myth" was part of a grand conspiracy, what were the reasons for starting it, and what benefits would there be for scientific researchers, food companies, and the U.S. government to continue to perpetuate this conspiracy?

Anyone with a basic scientific background can read the *Seven Countries* book[1] and understand that Dr. Keys presented a

1. Keys A, Aravanis C, Blackburn H, Buzina R, Djordjević BS, Dontas AS, Fidanza F, Karvonen MJ, Kimura N, Menotti A, Mohacek I, Nedeljković S, Puddu V,

balanced picture of the research and was, in fact, open minded about the biology behind the observations he and his colleagues made and the data they accumulated. In no way was Dr. Keys dogmatic in his descriptions or in his conclusions.

Furthermore, at the time of the Seven Countries Study, very little was understood about basic cholesterol and lipoprotein metabolism in the body.

If you look through the websites that mock Dr. Keys and his basic findings, it is obvious that each uses similar catch phrases, and there is little comprehensive knowledge of the sciences of nutrition and medicine evident in their criticisms.

Let's go back and concisely review Dr. Ancel Keys's life, career, and contributions to science and health.[2] A more thorough biography of Dr. Keys is currently being written by historian Dr. Sarah Tracy. Dr. Keys attended the University of California where he earned a B.A. in economics, an M.A. in zoology, and in 1930, a Ph.D. in oceanography and biology. Dr. Keys traveled to Denmark as a National Research Council Fellow to work with Dr. August Krogh, a Nobel Prize-winning physiologist, on the control of salt concentration in tissues of marine organisms. After this experience, Dr. Keys studied high-altitude physiology with Dr. Joseph Bancroft, a professor at King's College of Cambridge University. In 1938 Ancel Keys received a second Ph.D. from the University of Cambridge, England, and then was offered a position at the Harvard Fatigue Laboratory at Harvard University. One of his projects involved a six-month expedition to northern Chile to study the physiological adaptation to high altitude. This expedition climbed the Andes Mountains to Aguada Quilcha, a miners' village at 17,500 feet. It was on this trip that Dr. Keys donated a blood sample at 20,000 feet. This would register to be

Punsar S, Taylor HL, Van Buchem FSP. (1980) *Seven Countries. A multivariate analysis of death and coronary heart disease.* Cambridge, MA: Harvard University Press, ISBN: 0-674-80237-3, 381 pp.

2. Websites of the University of Minnesota and Division of Epidemiology and Community Health: http://www.epi.umn.edu/cvdepi

the blood sample taken at the highest altitude for many years.[3 4] After Harvard, Dr. Keys worked for less than a year at the Mayo Clinic in Rochester, Minnesota. Although his experiences at the Mayo were scientifically curtailed, he did have the good fortune of hiring Margaret Haney for a laboratory technician position. Margaret, who was from Minnesota, had received a bachelor's degree in chemistry from Wells College in upstate New York. Soon afterward, Ancel and Margaret were married and moved to Minneapolis for what would be their permanent home.

In 1939 Dr. Keys became a professor of physiology at the University of Minnesota, where he established the Laboratory of Physiological Hygiene in the School of Public Health. During World War II, Dr. Keys, because of his expertise in the physiology of extreme altitude, was asked to develop small, easily transportable packets of food that later were called K rations. After this Dr. Keys was appointed Special Assistant to the Secretary of War, and was involved in many different war-related projects. He evaluated emergency rations to be stored in life rafts, and because of his early research on the physiological adaptation to high altitude and cold temperatures, Dr. Keys advised the Army and Navy on warm clothing for extreme cold temperatures.[5] These were important contributions to the war effort. During the war Dr. Keys realized that many soldiers and civilians would suffer from starvation. Therefore, after a proposal was approved by the

3. Hoffman W. (1979) "Meet Monsieur Cholesterol" (Profile of world-renowned cardiovascular epidemiologist Ancel Keys). *Update* (University of Minnesota). http://mbbnet.umn.edu/hoff/hoff_ak.html
4. Documentary: *Health Revolutionary: The Life and Work of Ancel Keys*, University of Minnesota School of Public Health, c2002, Available at Andersen Library University Archives una105009 (Film 768). https://umedia.lib.umn.edu/node/88945?mode=
5. Report from the War Department to Ancel Keys - University of Minnesota Archives-Visited August 2014. Ancel B. Keys papers, Creator: Keys, Ancel Benjamin, 1904-2004; Extent: 2 boxes (0.45 cubic feet); Repository: University of Minnesota Libraries, Elmer L. Andersen Library, uar@umn.edu; Collection Number: uarc 738 https://www.lib.umn.edu/special/getting-archives

War Department, he began a study of the physiological changes that occur in humans during starvation. The participants in the study were 36 male conscientious objectors. The point of this study was to understand the basic physiological mechanisms that were in play during starvation, and to find the best way to treat a starving person from a medical and nutritional perspective. This information later became invaluable to doctors treating prisoners and starved civilians during and after World War II. Dr. Keys's studies on starvation led to the publication in 1950 of the two-volume monograph, *Biology of Human Starvation.*[6] This book, which included field observations obtained during World War II, is considered the definitive work on starvation. A concise article on the human starvation studies performed at the University of Minnesota was also published.[7] A newly published book by Todd Tucker chronicles the starvation studies performed at the University of Minnesota during World War II.[8] This book also describes Dr. Keys' early research career in detail.

After the war Dr. Keys turned his attention to the large number of men who were dying of heart attacks at a relatively young age. In 1947, Dr. Keys first studied local businessmen and administrators at the University of Minnesota, ages 39 to 60, because this was the age that many men were dying prematurely from coronary heart disease. If you view the documentary film on Dr. Ancel Keys on the University of Minnesota Library website,[9] it shows the men visiting Dr. Keys's lab for their annual physical checkups. These businessmen, in one way, were typical of men of the 1940s-1950s. They were well fed and slightly overweight. They were usually dressed in a suit. And they appeared to all

6. Keys A, Brožek J, Henschel A, Mickelsen O, Taylor HL. (1950) *The biology of human starvation.* (2 vols). Oxford, England: University of Minnesota Press. 1385 pp.
7. Keys A. (1946) Human Starvation and Its Consequences. *Journal of the American Dietetic Association* 22: 482-487.
8. Tucker T. (2006) *The Great Starvation Experiment - The Heroic Men Who Starved So That Millions Could Live.* New York: Free Press (Simon & Schuster).
9. Ancel Keys: A Brief Profile: https://www.youtube.com/watch?v=kOifkb4JlfY

smoke. But they were not typical of most American men in another important way. They were, for the most part, from the upper socioeconomic class found in the urban St. Paul-Minneapolis area. Twenty-five percent were the presidents or vice-presidents of large businesses.

Dr. Keys's seminal observation was that the men who had heart attacks tended to have higher concentrations of cholesterol in their blood. What is truly outstanding about this study is that it is one of the first of its kind. Medicine was just entering the age of true modern advances. The first antibiotic was used during World War II. The science of nutrition was still in the period known mainly for the discovery of vitamins. Little was known about why or how heart attacks occurred in middle-aged humans who otherwise appeared to be healthy men and, in lesser numbers, healthy women. Although this was an important project, the Minnesota business and professional men study was limited because the particular group of men examined and followed was not representative of a wide cross section of American men, and also the number of participants was small. However, Dr. Keys learned from this study, and it was instrumental in guiding him during the development of the much larger Seven Countries Study.

It is beneficial to examine the research paper for this first diet-coronary heart disease study as it gives insights into Dr. Keys's propensity for experimental detail and balanced viewpoint. The paper was published in 1963 after the 15-year follow-up was completed.[10]

10. Keys A, Blackburn HW, Taylor HL, Brožek J, Anderson JT, Simonson E. (1963) Coronary heart disease among Minnesota business and professional men followed fifteen years. *Circulation* 28: 381–395. http://www.ncbi.nlm.nih.gov/pubmed/?term=14059458

Let's revisit important parts of this early study in Dr. Keys's own words. He wrote:

> The main purpose of this report is to compare, in respect to the measurements considered here, the pre-disease characteristics of the men who developed coronary heart disease with the contemporary characteristics of their fellows who did not develop the disease.
>
> The men in the present study are not a statistical sample of American men or even of middle-aged men in Minnesota. They were drawn from men in the upper socioeconomic class in the metropolitan area of St. Paul-Minneapolis; one fourth are (or were) presidents or vice-presidents of substantial corporations; more than half of the group were college men. This is a native-born and educated group, almost all with ancestral origins in the British Isles, the Scandinavian countries (mainly Norway and Sweden), and Germany.

Serum cholesterol was the only parameter that was statistically significant in this study.

> The incidence of coronary heart disease tended to be higher among men above the median at first examination in relative weight, body fatness, systolic and diastolic blood pressure, and serum cholesterol concentration but these segregations were not statistically significant except with serum cholesterol, which was associated with $p < 0.001$.

But some men did not have high cholesterol and still suffered heart attacks.

> The general conclusion seems warranted, then, that men who develop coronary heart disease in spite of having relatively low serum cholesterol values are men who tend to be at the upper extremes of blood pressure or relative body weight, or both.

My conclusions from reading this paper:

This is a very good research paper even if the men studied were not representative of all American men in the 1950s. Dr. Keys and his colleagues described their methods exquisitely, they reported their findings in a balanced way, and they reported that the study was not representative and that it was too small.

Then the authors compared their results on diet and coronary heart disease to the results of several other similar studies being carried on about the same time.

There were no wild hypotheses. There was no bombastic language. There was no indication that a zealot was window dressing his results.

From this rather small study, Dr. Keys and his colleagues went on to design a much larger study that would search for the answers to what was causing massive numbers of heart attacks in American men in the 1940s and 1950s. This larger study, which officially began in 1958, later became known as the Seven Countries Study.

2.

HOW THE SEVEN COUNTRIES STUDY WAS CONCEIVED

When Dr. Ancel Keys and his colleagues wrote the *Seven Countries* book (published in 1980),[1] they seemed to follow the strategy of writing "Just the facts" from this multi-country study and interpreted the data as best they could without exaggerated speculation. However, the exciting and much more interesting human story of how Dr. Keys came upon his theory that diet and blood cholesterol were responsible for the high rates of coronary artery disease (CHD) in some populations is not in *Seven Countries*. In fact, the interesting story of how he developed his ideas and how he "discovered" the Mediterranean diet were presented in the first few chapters of the third cookbook that he and his wife, Margaret, wrote in 1975. They had first published *Eat Well and Stay Well in 1959*,[2] and then revised it and released it in 1975 as *How to Eat Well and Stay Well the Mediterranean Way.*[3]

1. Keys A. *et al.* (1980) *Seven Countries. A multivariate analysis of death and coronary heart disease....(full reference in chapter 1)*
2. Keys A, Keys M. (1959) *Eat Well and Stay Well*. Garden City, New York: Doubleday & Company.

The 1975 book is rather hard to find nowadays. I could not find it in either the Rutgers University or New York Public Library systems. When I tried to buy it on Amazon and other websites, it was listed at over $300 for a used copy. However, if you find this book in a used bookstore, buy it, not because of a windfall profit, but because it is surely a gem of a book. I finally found it in a local library in New Jersey that seems to specialize in cookbooks!

In the author's preface, Dr. Keys and Margaret give the background for the book and graciously thank all the scientists, physicians, and friends who were involved in the work and who helped them in their travels around the globe in search for the causes of coronary heart disease. They write that the book was the result of 25 years of research by them with the help of hundreds of coworkers and friends. No where is it stated that their endeavors were due to a singular enterprise. They give ample credit to many others who contributed to their story.

In chapter 1, "Introduction-Why and How," Dr. Keys and Margaret explain, in a relatively short chapter, how the idea about diet being an important component in the onset of coronary heart disease was hatched, how it progressed slowly at first, and then, how the concept was formally presented and studied under the well-planned structure of the Seven Countries Study. Anyone who has heard the invectives that claim that the diet-cholesterol-coronary heart disease theory was a conspiracy put forth by Dr. Ancel Keys can't possibly believe this claim after reading the story of how the ideas coalesced among Dr. Keys and his colleagues.

How to Eat Well and Stay Well the Mediterranean Way, which is a combination who-done-it mystery and health/cookbook, was written before there was any controversy concerning the fat and cholesterol hypothesis, and therefore, the detailed descriptions of how their ideas were conceived were written without any sense of defending a core idea. In fact, what comes across in chapter 1 is

3. Keys A, Keys M. (1975) *How to Eat Well and Stay Well the Mediterranean Way*. Garden City, New York: Doubleday & Company.

a sense of wonder at how a meandering course led to one of the most important discoveries in modern medicine. And it is hard for us to realize that at the beginning of their journey, no one had any idea about what caused coronary heart disease, or that simple changes in lifestyle could protect against coronary heart disease, or that the opposite was possible too–changes could also enhance its ghastly effects.

Although Dr. Keys had been a successful and well-known scientist since the 1930s and had been involved in a variety of studies, including measuring cholesterol in blood in several smaller studies, the Seven Countries story really began in February 1952, when the Keyses first traveled to Naples, Italy, to study the role of diet in coronary heart disease.[4] They had been living in England as part of a Fulbright Fellowship, and they had been invited to the University of Naples by Professor Gino Bergami, who mentioned that cases of coronary heart disease were very rare in Naples.

On their visit to Naples, the Keyses were going to follow-up on the dual observations made by local physicians that the local Neapolitan diet was low in fat and that there were few cases of coronary heart disease among the common people of the city. The Keyses did, in fact, find this to be true, and found that the men they studied in Naples had an average cholesterol level of 165, compared to the average level of 230 that was usually observed in Minnesota. Later on that year, the Keyses visited Spain for the purpose of observing the eating habits of the people in several villages there. They observed a similar situation concerning the foods eaten and the good health of the people living in these villages. The Keyses' trips to these two Mediterranean countries were fairly casual, but the observations they made had a great impact on them, and these observations pointed to the hypothesis that the diet consumed in these communities, at the time, appeared to protect against coronary heart disease.

4. Keys A, Keys M. (1975) Ibid., page 2.

Although not originally conceived in this way, the start of the Seven Countries Study was to be accomplished in two stages. First, there was a period of pre-studies (1952-56) that were carried out to determine whether a full study could be implemented in such a way. After all, this was the first time such a study would be attempted, and it was not known whether investigations like this, carried out in seven different countries, would be even possible. The pre-studies involved Dr. Keys and his wife, Margaret, a few colleagues from Minnesota, and physicians and technicians from the countries being studied. It was during this early period when Dr. Keys sought out reliable colleagues who could help in the study. In many ways, these colleagues also sought Dr. Keys out. In fact, the coalescing of the principal researchers was quite magical. Possibly, the investigators in the participating countries had met Dr. Keys and were captivated by his energy and ideas. It was at this time–when the first collaborations were starting–that the seeds of success for the Seven Countries Study were planted. However, the Seven Countries Study did not officially begin until fall 1958 after a formal grant application was submitted in 1957 and subsequently funded (See time line).

In the spring of 1954, the year I was born, the Keyses returned to Naples a second time to continue their studies. They brought with them several other investigators, including the prestigious American cardiologist, Paul Dudley White, who was later to serve as President Eisenhower's cardiologist. They extended their studies to several other sites in Italy, including Cagliari, on the island of Sardinia, and the northern city of Bologna, known for having a richer cuisine than the other locations in Italy. Their previous findings concerning the fat content of the diet and blood cholesterol concentrations held up in these locations as well.

The year 1954 also saw the beginning of a collaboration between Dr. Keys and Dr. Noboru Kimura, a young heart doctor from Japan.[5] A monthlong visit to Japan by Dr. Keys and his team informally confirmed the widely reported, but unsubstantiated claims, that Japanese men, who were fairly heavy smokers, had very low rates of coronary heart disease. By 1956, a fair sized pre-study was started by Dr. Kimura in Fukuoka, Japan, a city with surrounding farming villages and also a nearby U.S. military base.

Informal pilot studies also commenced in Hawaii, where men of European ancestry who consumed a fairly typical American diet could be compared to men of Japanese ancestry, who still followed a basically Japanese diet.

The results were startling: the Japanese in Fukuoka, Japan, and those Japanese in Hawaii who adhered to a native Japanese diet, had blood cholesterol concentrations of about 160, but the white Americans in Hawaii had cholesterol levels similar to the white men Ancel Keys had studied in Minnesota.[6] This led to an interesting, yet unique conclusion at the time. The conclusion was that high cholesterol and high rates of coronary heart disease were not directly related to climate! Sounds funny now, but this really was considered a possibility at the time. Although these studies created excitement in the medical community, their small size indicated that a more definitive study with adequate numbers of study subjects and more sophisticated survey methods were needed.

In 1956 Dr. Keys was visited in Minnesota by Professor Martti Karvonen of the Institute of Occupational Health in Helsinki, Finland. Dr. Keys had met him earlier at the first Food and Agriculture Organization meeting in Rome. Dr. Karvonen suggested that Finland might provide a contrast to the diet and coronary heart disease observed in Japan and Italy. Dr. Keys and his team traveled to Finland and the first Finnish area they sampled was East Karelia, where they found very high rates of coronary heart disease among the men. The average blood cholesterol concentration was a shocking 260, compared to the

5. Keys A, Keys M. (1975) Ibid., Page 7.
6. Keys A, Keys M. (1975) Ibid., page 8.

230 Dr. Keys had consistently measured among men in Minnesota. When he saw what the Finns ate, however, the likely cause of their high cholesterol values became apparent. Dr. Keys stated that he, "...watched in disbelief to see some of them take slabs of cheese the size of slices of sandwich bread, smear them a quarter of an inch deep with butter and eat them, with a beer, as an after-sauna snack."[7]

In 1957 Dr. Keys formulated a design for the formal Seven Countries Study and conducted a pilot run with a team of scientists he had assembled with common interests in cultural differences in diet and heart disease. They tested survey methods and responses in the village of Nicotera, near the toe of the Italian boot, and they also visited several villages on the island of Crete. The blood cholesterol levels were very low (160) in Nicotera because of the extremely low fat intake of its inhabitants. Below is a photograph of Dr. Keys in a street in Nicotera, Italy, discussing a pressing issue with Drs. Flaminio Fidanza, Martti Karvonen, and Noboru Kimura.[8]

7. Keys A, Keys M. (1975) Ibid., page 11.
8. Photograph courtesy of Dr. Henry Blackburn, Division of Epidemiology and Community Medicine, University of Minnesota.

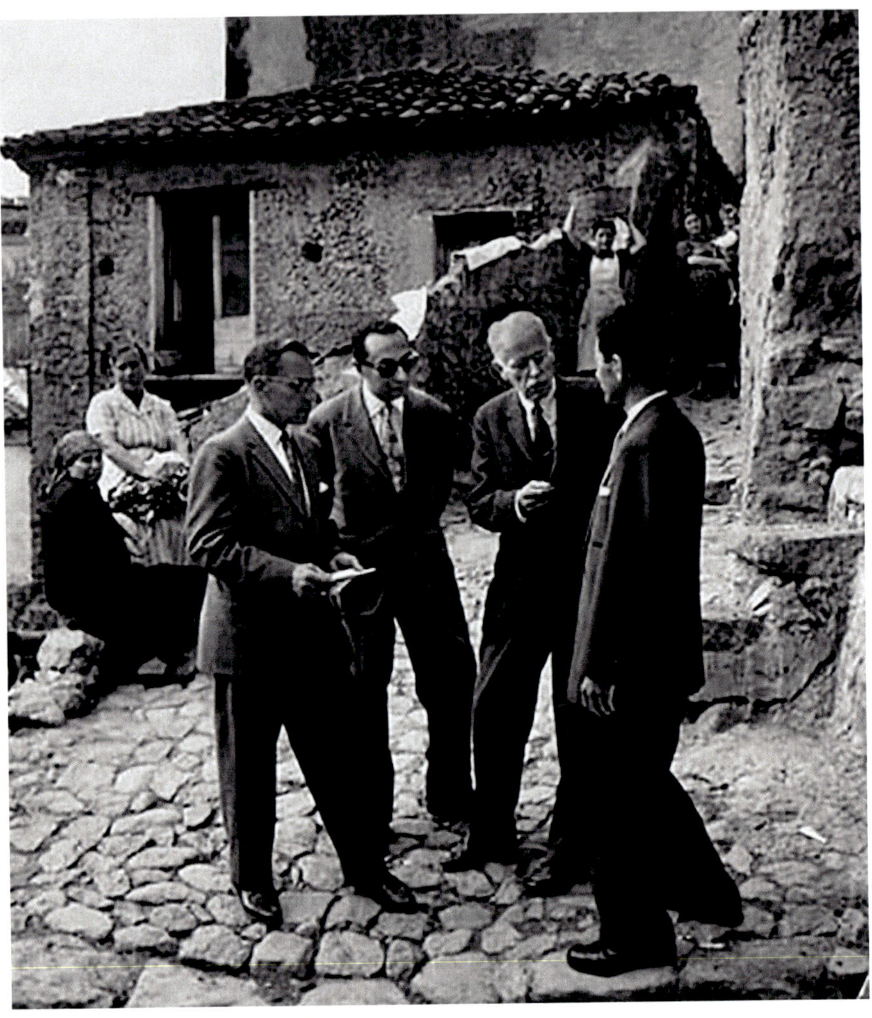

Drs. Ancel Keys, Flaminio Fidanza, Martti Karvonen, and Noboru Kimura on a street in Nicotera, Italy. Photograph courtesy of Dr. Henry Blackburn, University of Minnesota. See hundreds of photographs at: http://www.epi.umn.edu/cvdepi/multimedia/photographs/

Crete was especially interesting because the fat intake was relatively high there. But because most of the fat consumed was olive oil, the cholesterol concentrations in the blood of the men of Crete were below 200. In the 1950s the foods on Crete were served usually drenched in olive oil. Butter and milk were not consumed. Meat was only consumed once or twice per week. Some farmers had the habit of drinking wine glasses of pure olive oil for breakfast![9] Although roughly one third of the calories consumed on Crete were from fat, the rates of coronary heart disease were extremely low. This was an early sign that it was the type of fat that was important in influencing the cholesterol levels of blood, and not total fat intake per se. Dr. Keys said that this observation strongly influenced his thinking.[10]

All of what had been experienced on these relatively short trips by Dr. Keys and his staff amounted to a feasibility study for a much larger study. After the grant application was favorably reviewed and then funded, the plans went forward to start a well-designed study that would measure blood cholesterol, other characteristics, and rates of coronary heart disease, using state-of-the-art methods,[11] such as electrocardiography, in different populations throughout the world. It would also measure in precise ways the dietary intakes of subjects in the different regions. In the fall of 1958, an official study was commenced that would eventually became known as the Seven Countries Study. There would eventually be about 13,000 men enrolled in seven countries, with some countries providing several distinct geographical locations to be studied.

One must remember that the Seven Countries Study was started before statin drugs had been discovered. Therefore, there was a great deal of emphasis on stopping the onset and progression of coronary heart disease, which was already a scourge of Western populations. As discussed in later chapters

9. Keys A, Keys M. (1975) Ibid., page 17.
10. Henry Blackburn interview of Ancel Keys, Jan. 9, 1991, at the offices and labs inside Stadium Gate 27, the longtime home of the University of Minnesota Laboratory of Physiological Hygiene. http://www.epi.umn.edu/cvdepi/video/henry-blackburn-interviews-ancel-keys/
11. Blackburn, H. Field Methods for the New Discipline of CVD Epidemiology. http://www.epi.umn.edu/cvdepi/the-research/methods/

of this book, dietary recommendations changed in Finland as a result of the Seven Countries Study, leading to a significant decrease in coronary heart disease. But changes occurred in the opposite direction, too. As Europe recovered from the drastic effects of World War II, the diet of many Europeans began to become richer in terms of meat and dairy products. This had the effect of slowly increasing coronary heart disease where before there had been almost none. The Mediterranean diet would become less “Mediterranean” in several of the cohorts during the follow-up periods to the Seven Countries Study.

3.

IMPLEMENTING THE SEVEN COUNTRIES STUDY

One of the major invectives media nutrition writers hurl at Dr. Ancel Keys is that he intentionally left out data from other countries that would have decimated the strength of his main observation that coronary heart disease was correlated with blood cholesterol concentrations across the seven countries. This criticism is just nonsense and, in fact, chronologically and historically untrue. A later study of 40 countries completely supported Dr. Keys's observations in the Seven Countries Study and I will address the results of this study in this chapter. If you read the comments of the investigators who were associated with the Seven Countries Study, there is no indication that subsets of data were eliminated from the study.

At the time of Dr. Keys's 100th birthday, Professor Mario Mancini of the Universitfldi Napoli, Naples, Italy, and Dr. Jerry Stamler, who led the MRFIT study, wrote of their early associations with Dr. Keys and how the results from the Seven

Countries Study were important in the establishment of high blood cholesterol as a risk factor for coronary heart disease.[1]

Dr. Mancini described how, in 1954, Dr. Keys organized a meeting in Naples, to discuss with leading investigators from across Europe a study that would investigate the role of diet and lifestyle on the incidence of coronary heart disease in middle-aged males across a spectrum of countries. The countries to be enrolled included Finland, Greece, Italy, Japan, the Netherlands, United States, and Yugoslavia.

Dr. Mancini is now one of the most respected physicians in Italy. As a young doctor in 1957 he was invited by Dr. Keys to be part of the international team that performed a pilot study in Nicotera, Calabria, a region in southern Italy where coronary heart disease was "non-existent." Dr. Mancini goes on to highlight Dr. Keys's role in combating coronary heart disease through primary prevention rather than by treatment after the fact. In this article from 2004 Professor Mancini also commented, "Ancel Keys and his wife Margaret were highly impressed by the eating patterns of the Mediterranean cohorts participating in the SCS and therefore decided to write the book that became a best seller, '*Eat Well and Stay Well*' where great merit is given to the Mediterranean diet for the prevention of coronary heart disease and for longevity (9, 10). The ages that its authors have now reached (100 yrs Ancel and 95 Margaret Keys) lend support to their evaluation."

As reviewed in chapter 2 of this book, the motivation to investigate the role of diet in the development of coronary heart disease is most clearly presented in, *How to Eat Well and Stay Well the Mediterranean Way.*[2] If you read the early chapters in

1. Mancini M, Stamler J. (2004) Diet for preventing cardiovascular diseases: Light from Ancel Keys, Distinguished Centenarian Scientist. *Nutr Metab Cardiovasc Dis* 14: 52-57. http://www.ncbi.nlm.nih.gov/pubmed/?term=15053164
2. Keys A, Keys M. (1975) *How to Stay Well and Eat Well the Mediterranean Way.* Garden City, New York: Doubleday & Company.

Seven Countries, Dr. Keys elaborated on how the different groups of men were chosen and described the methods that were used to study them. The cohorts selected were men, 40 to 59 years old, usually from a well-defined area where the total population of men were asked to participate in the study. The response rate for most of the groups asked to participate was over 90%, which is an excellent recruitment rate. Although seven countries were involved, more than one area was studied within most of the countries, so the total number of cohorts equaled 16, of which 11 were from rural regions. The geographical locations of the cohorts are shown in the following figure.[3]

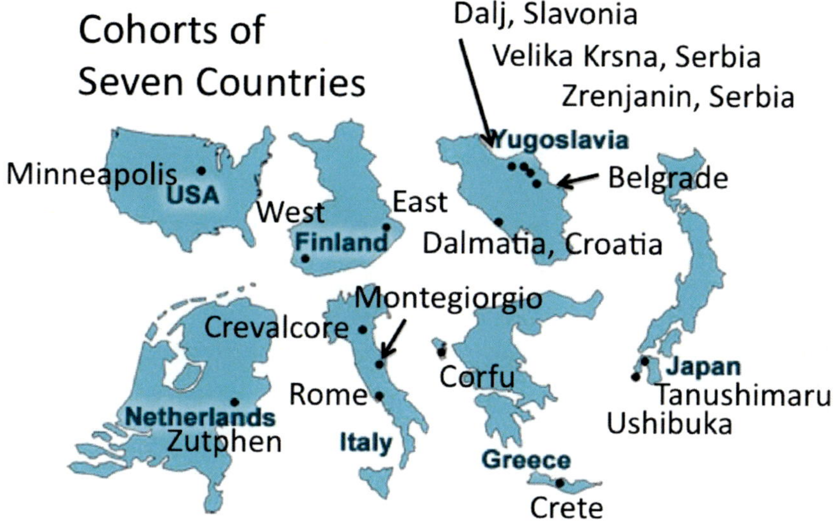

Cohorts studied in the Seven Countries Study. Figure adapted from http://sevencountriesstudy.com

The particular countries used in the study were chosen because a group of experienced researchers was available to participate in

3. Figure adapted from Seven Countries website http://sevencountriesstudy.com/about-the-study/countries

the country and the countries represented a wide range of dietary intakes. The areas within each country were chosen because they represented defined areas with distinct diet contrasts and a stable populations of men. Rural farming areas with men of low mobility were considered ideal locations as the investigators wished to perform follow-up examinations at regular intervals.[4] The group of men recruited in the United States were comprised of railroad workers, both office workers and more active switchmen, from the area outlined by the Twin Cities (Minneapolis and St. Paul), St. Louis, San Francisco, and Seattle.[5] (The railroad workers are described in greater detail in a later chapter in this book.) To make a direct comparison with the American cohort, a similar group of railroad workers was identified and recruited in Italy.

The purpose of reviewing how the study was started is to show, that for the time period, this was a brilliant, out-of-the-box study that was conceived by a curious scientist who wished to find an answer to a serious medical mystery. One has to remember that the study was started in the 1950s, before the advent of personal computers, Excel spreadsheets, the internet, cell phones, and commercial jet aircraft. But what was especially amazing about the Seven Countries Study was that it was started by Ancel Keys through his contacts with many of the top physicians and scientists throughout the world, and anyone who has worked with such high-energy individuals knows how hard it is to convince them to commit to a large project. In a way, Ancel Keys's true gift was to persuade these distinguished scientists to buy into and commit to the Seven Countries Study.

Reviews of each country and descriptions of the main colleagues involved can be found in *Seven Countries,*[6] by Ancel

4. Henry Blackburn interview of Ancel Keys, Jan. 9, 1991, at the University of Minnesota Laboratory of Physiological Hygiene (Stadium Gate 27). http://www.epi.umn.edu/cvdepi/video/henry-blackburn-interviews-ancel-keys/
5. Blackburn H. (1995) Chapter 6 "The U.S. Railroad Study," In: *On the trail of heart attacks in Seven Countries.* Middleborough, MA: The Country Press Inc.

Keys and colleagues; *How to Eat Well and Stay Well the Mediterranean Way,* by Ancel and Margaret Keys; *The Seven Countries Study: A scientific adventure in cardiovascular disease epidemiology;*[7] and, *On the Trail of Heart Attacks in Seven Countries,*[8] by Henry Blackburn.

The very beginnings of the Seven Countries Study were recalled by Dr. Blackburn in his book and are paraphrased here: September, 1958 – Dr. Blackburn arrived in Zagreb in Tito's Yugoslavia. He traveled to Dalmatia (Croatia), populated with both farmers and fishermen, to participate with the study group carrying out the clinical examinations there. He remained until mid October and then moved onto Slavonia (Croatia), where there were mostly farmers. Dr. Blackburn administered electrocardiography exams to study participants in order to determine whether any participants had suffered previous heart attacks. On November 4, Dr. Blackburn departed Yugoslavia and on his way home to Minnesota, he needed to travel in a zigzag pattern through Italy, Austria, and England, because direct travel at the time was not possible. Recruitment in Yugoslavia was above 95%, meaning that 95% of a targeted group agreed to participate in the study. Major collaborators in Yugoslavia were the nutritional scientist Ratko Buzina and cardiologist Ivan Mohacek in Zagreb, and Professor Bozidar and cardiologist Drejko Nedeljkovic in Belgrade.

Also in 1958, investigations in southern Japan launched as an official wing of the Seven Countries Study. Dr. Noboru Kimura of Japan had visited Minnesota in 1952 and stayed in close contact with Dr. Keys. Dr. Kimura had helped out in the clinical pre-

6. Keys A. et al. (1980) Seven Countries...(full reference in chapter 1)
7. Kromhout D, Menotti A, Blackburn H (Eds). (1994) The Seven Countries Study: *The Seven Countries Study: A scientific adventure in cardiovascular disease epidemiology.* Brouwer Offset b.v., Utrecht, ISBN 90-6960-048-x, 219 pp. The entire text can be found on line at: http://sevencountriesstudy.com/study-findings/publications
8. Blackburn H. (1995) On the trail of heart attacks in Seven Countries. Middleborough, MA: The Country Press Inc.

studies in Italy and Crete in 1957. In 1958 Dr. Kimura commenced a cohort of the Seven Countries Study in the southern farming village of Tanushimaru, Japan. Later on, Dr. Kimura initiated a second Japanese cohort in the nearby fishing village of Ushibuka, Japan. One of the aims of the Japanese wing was to study the differences in inhabitants of a fishing village versus a farming village.

In the United States, Dr. Henry Longstreet Taylor, professor at the Laboratory of Physiological Hygiene in Minnesota, began the U.S. cohort of the Seven Countries Study as part of the examination of U.S. railroad men (USRR Study). Dr. Henry Blackburn's career began at the University of Minnesota in 1953 as an intern with Dr. Taylor on the USRR Study. This part of the study will be discussed in greater detail in chapter 8.

In 1959, studies in East and West Finland joined the Seven Countries Study. Finland was chosen because both Ancel Keys and Martti Karvonen thought the dichotomies found in East Finland–hard-working farmers and loggers who appeared hardy and strong, but in reality, suffered from very high rates of coronary heart disease–would provide important clues to the causes of coronary heart disease. In the same country, the people of West Finland appeared less prone to coronary heart disease, possibly due to living closer to the sea coast and the consumption of a diet high in fish and marine oils. One interesting experience that the Seven Countries Study visiting investigators were subjected to was a classic Finnish country sauna.[9] Dr. Blackburn relates how he, along with all the native medical staff, entered a sauna and were exposed to "a searing blast of hot air beyond any previous experience," only to be exposed a few seconds later to an even a hotter blast of heat. Then, when they could not take the heat any longer, each person burst out of the sauna and ran down the dock and dove into the ice cold lake water. After recovering while sitting around a campfire with beer and

9. Blackburn H. (1995) Ibid., page 69.

food, Dr. Blackburn felt relaxed and amazed that he had survived this "sacred" Finnish tradition! In chapter 5, I cover the great success experienced by the Finns when, because of the findings of the Seven Countries Study, they adjusted their diet and other risk factors and lowered their very high rates of coronary heart disease.

By 1960, additional arms of the Seven Countries Study were ready to come onboard. In 1960 and 1961 cohorts of men were started in Ushibuka, Japan; Crevalcore and Montegiogio, Italy; Zutphen, Netherlands; and Crete and Corfu, Greece. In Japan, Dr. Kimura started a second Japanese cohort in the fishing village of Ushibuka, Japan. In Italy, the town of Crevalcore in the Po Valley, about an hour north of Bologna, was chosen because of the richness, including a high intake of fat, of the northern Italian food served there. The other Italian area, the villages surrounding Montegiogio, was situated on the Adriatic coast of Italy. The Italian colleagues that were instrumental early on were Dr. Flaminio Fidanza, who had first met Dr. Ancel Keys when he visited Naples in 1952, and Dr. Vittorio Puddu, who helped the Seven Countries Study investigators obtain access to Italian hospitals and who recruited young physician-helpers. One of those helpers was a young physician, Dr. Alessandro Menotti, who would turn out to be one of the coleaders of the Seven Countries Study during its second 25 years. Another helper was Dr. Mario Mancini, who was an early visitor to the Laboratory of Physiological Hygiene in Minnesota and who helped in some of the pre-studies.

A cohort for the Seven Countries Study was established in the Netherlands because the diet there represented a middle ground between the Mediterranean diets of southern Europe and the high meat, low fiber diets of northern Europe. The Dutch scientists chose Zutphen for the site, and, except for the reading of patient electrocardiograms by Dr. Henry Blackburn, who traveled to the Netherlands expressly for this purpose, all the work was performed by Dutch clinicians. Dr. Van Buchem led the study in the Netherlands in the early years, and was superseded in 1978 by Dr. Daan Kromhout, a Dutch nutritionist, who later became one of the coleaders of the Seven Countries Study along with Dr. Alessandro Menotti and Dr. Henry Blackburn. Dr. Daan Kromhout proved crucial to the continuation of the Seven Countries Study through its 50th year by obtaining adequate funding from European resources. Dr. Kromhout also specialized in studies investigating the role of the intake of fish in protecting against coronary heart disease.[10]

Crete and Corfu, Greece–The early visits during the pre-studies to Crete in the extreme south and Corfu, in the northwest, greatly influenced Dr. Ancel Keys, and official cohorts for the Seven Countries Study were recruited in these locations in 1960 and 1961. The on-site Greek collaborators included Christ Aravanis of Athens, who provided independent funding for large portions of the Greek studies, and Anastasios Dontas, a young investigator, who Dr. Blackburn stated, "provided the glue between Greece and Minnesota, professionally and collegially." Anyone interested in this part of the Seven Countries Study story should read Dr. Blackburn's book, *On the Trail of Heart Attacks in Seven Countries*, published in 1995. The start of the Rome railroad study and the remaining cohorts that were started in Serbia from 1962 to 1964 are also described in Dr. Blackburn's book.

In order to counter the arguments of media personalities that Dr. Keys gerrymandered the results by leaving out data from certain countries, I would like to discuss at this time a later study that was comprised of national health statistics data from 40 countries.[11]

10. Kromhout D. (2002) Chapter 2.2, "Diet and Coronary Heart Disease in the Zutphen Study," pp 71-84. In: Kromhout D, Menotti A, Blackburn H (Eds). Prevention of coronary heart disease. Diet, lifestyle and risk factors in the Seven Countries Study. Kluwer Academic Publishers, Boston.
11. Artaud-Wild SM, Connor SL, Sexton G and Connor WE. (1993) Differences in coronary mortality can be explained by differences in cholesterol and

The authors of this study (referred to as the Connor Study) gathered health statistics and food intake (40 dietary variables) data from forty countries that spanned many levels of socioeconomic status. The authors also used a simple Cholesterol-Saturated Fat Index that allowed for comparisons using the combined dietary intakes of cholesterol and saturated fat. When the data were analyzed, coronary heart disease mortality was highly correlated with the Cholesterol-Saturated Fat Index across all of the countries, except for France and Finland. This correlation is shown in the figure presented below.

saturated fat intakes in 40 countries but not in France and Finland. A paradox. *Circulation* 88: 2771-2779 http://circ.ahajournals.org/content/88/6/2771.long

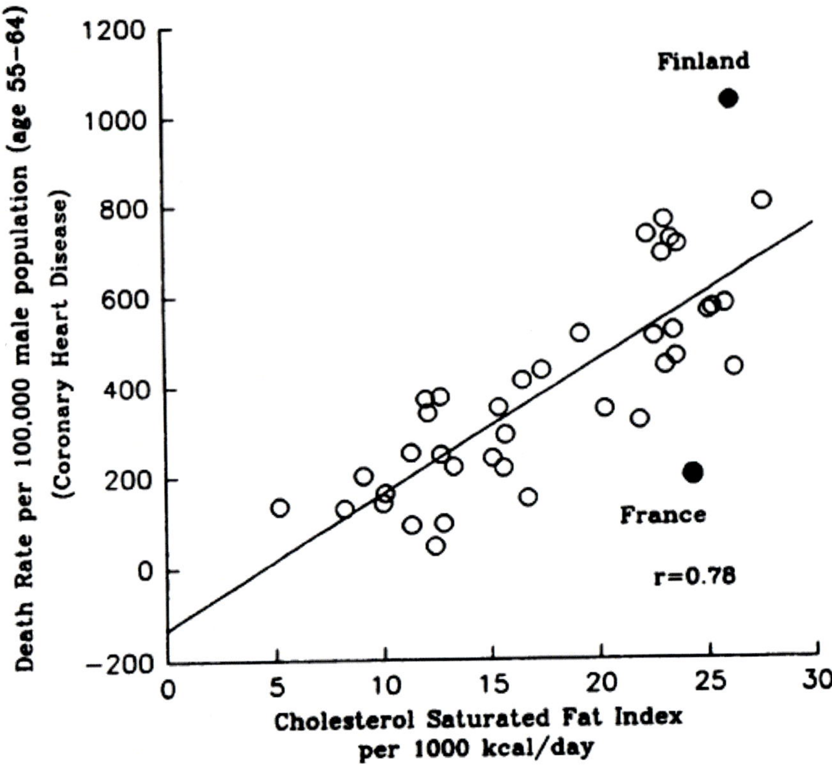

Figure 2A from Astaud-Wild et al. (1993) *Circulation* 88: 2771-2779. r=0.76 is the correlation coefficient (a measure of how good the data fits the line). Each circle represents data from a different country.

Although all of the data were derived from national health statistics, and this type of data varies from country to country based upon level of medical sophistication, the wide range of data accumulated allows a moderate level of confidence concerning the results. The figure shows that deaths from coronary heart disease were highly correlated with the intake of saturated fat and cholesterol over 38 countries. France was off the correlation line due to the fact that there was much less coronary heart disease for a high Cholesterol-Saturated Fat Index, and Finland was off the line because there was much more coronary heart disease than expected for the high Cholesterol-Saturated Fat Index value that characterized Finnish intake of fat and cholesterol. The authors noted these apparent abnormalities and called them a paradox. They analyzed the dietary data for these two countries and found that Finns consumed much more milk and butterfat (fat from milk, cream, cheese, and butter) than the French. On the other hand, the French consumed more vegetables and vegetable oils than the Finns. Interestingly, the Connor study pointed to milk fat, especially butter, as a potent pro-coronary heart disease dietary factor. The results of this study completely replicated the physical measurements directly collected by Dr. Keys and his colleagues in the Seven Countries Study.

The Connor Study even observed a similar paradox as was observed by Keys. In the Seven Countries Study there was a large disparity between Finland and Crete, which had widely different rates of coronary heart disease at similar fat intakes. In the Connor study, there was a large disparity between Finland and France, which had widely different rates of coronary heart disease at similar fat intakes. Of course, as discussed in many scientific articles, these disparities were probably due to the protective effects of the Mediterranean diet in Crete and France. Overall, the Connor Study closely replicated the results of the earlier Seven Countries Study, but it did so using data from 40 countries. This study blows apart the singular criticism of the Seven Countries Study that Ancel Keys did not include data from other countries and thus he altered the results concerning the roles of cholesterol and saturated fat in the development of coronary heart disease. Furthermore, we must ask the question, why would Ancel Keys alter the results? The Connor Study definitely supported the results obtained in the Seven Countries Study, and my final conclusion must be that, in contrast to the recent wild utterances of the nutrition media zealots, Dr. Ancel Keys was an accurate and truthful scientist.

4.

A CLOSER LOOK AT SEVEN COUNTRIES

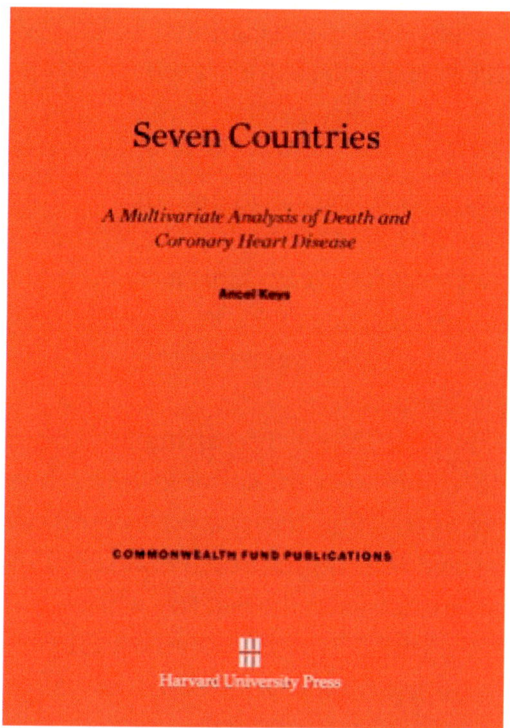

Cover of *Seven Countries*, by Ancel Keys and colleagues. (1980) Harvard University Press.

The study that pointed to saturated fat intake as a consistent association with coronary disease rates and burden in whole populations was the Seven Countries Study that was directed by Dr. Ancel Keys, a renowned physiologist who used epidemiology as another tool in an extensive armamentarium to scientifically study the increased rates of coronary heart disease among several populations, including the United States. This was a massive study that followed 12,763 men, aged 40-59, from seven countries with wide contrasts in traditional diet: Finland, Greece, Italy, Japan, the Netherlands, the United States, and Yugoslavia. The overall findings (from many published articles) of these studies, including the 10-year follow-up, were published in a book, *Seven Countries* by Ancel Keys and colleagues (1980).[1]

Before reviewing the major findings of the Seven Countries Study, I would like to take you on a short walk through the mysterious history of coronary heart disease in men in the United States. The surge in interest in this topic took place in the late 1940s and early 1950s, when middle-aged American men who looked healthy started to have heart attacks in astronomically large numbers. Researchers at the time began investigations into why these heart attacks were happening.

Interestingly, the Seven Countries Study was stimulated by the basic observation that blue-collar workers suffered fewer heart attacks than white-collar workers. But the reason for this was unknown. Dr. Keys hypothesized that high serum cholesterol was associated with higher heart attack rates in healthy white-collar workers, but this hypothesis, which was considered radical by many prominent scientists at the time, required extraordinary supportive data in order to show cause and effect.

Even scientists who accepted that blood cholesterol might be involved, also thought that the development of coronary heart disease resulted from multifactorial causes. Therefore, Dr. Keys's overall strategy was to perform a cross-cultural survey and investigate as many relevant factors as possible, including diet, blood pressure, occupation, and everything else that seemed pertinent.

As discussed above, researchers realized that the causes of coronary heart disease were multifactorial, but the factor that was probably blamed the most (by researchers and officials) at the time was serum cholesterol (and the intake of fat, especially saturated fat, in the diet). This was the case because additional

1. Keys A, Aravanis C, Blackburn H, Buzina R, Djordjević BS, Dontas AS, Fidanza F, Karvonen MJ, Kimura N, Menotti A, Mohacek I, Nedeljković S, Puddu V, Punsar S, Taylor HL, Van Buchem FSP. (1980) *Seven Countries. A multivariate analysis of death and coronary heart disease.* Cambridge, MA: Harvard University Press, ISBN: 0-674-80237-3, 381 pp.

studies, especially laboratory-controlled diet studies that were initiated at the same time, indicated that high intakes of saturated fat did, in fact, increase serum cholesterol. Focusing on blood cholesterol was also helped by the fact that the measurement of blood cholesterol concentration was fairly easy to perform in the laboratory.

However, if you read Ancel Keys's *Seven Countries* all the way through, you will find a balanced view of the fat/cholesterol hypothesis presented by the author. Right in the beginning of the book, Dr. Keys stated that there were observations in certain data sets he could not explain. And one of the major findings that appeared at the time was that serum cholesterol was particularly associated with coronary heart disease primarily at the higher concentrations of serum cholesterol. One caveat here, as discussed later in this chapter, is that the data presented in *Seven Countries* was only the 10-year follow-up data. Therefore, a very high blood cholesterol concentration was associated with the development of coronary heart disease during the relatively short 10-year follow-up period. After many more years of follow-up, and when larger data sets were analyzed and more definitive results were obtained, the consensus among researchers in the cholesterol-coronary heart disease field was (and still is) that blood cholesterol concentration is a continuously graded risk factor without a threshold point.

Significant Observations from *Seven Countries*

Now I wish to present the most interesting results from *Seven Countries*, by Dr. Keys and his colleagues. Below are a series of original figures and tables that I copied from the book taken from my bookshelf. There are over 120 figures of data and pages and pages of tables in *Seven Countries*. Therefore, these represent only a small percentage of the data contained within *Seven Countries*.

The figures below were selected and reproduced or copied from Ancel Keys's book.[2]

Title Page

Seven Countries – A Multivariate Analysis of Death and Coronary Heart Disease

Ancel Keys

with Christ Aravanis, Henry Blackburn, Ratko Buzini, B.S. Djordjevic, A.S. Dontas, Flaminio Fidanza, Martii J. Karvonen, Noboru Kimura, Alessandro Menotti, Ivan Mohacek, S. Nedeljkovic, Vittorio Puddu, Sven Punsar, Henry L. Taylor, and F.S.P. van Buchem

A Commonwealth Fund Book

Harvard University Press, Cambridge, Massachusetts and London, England 1980

2. Keys A. et al. (1980) *Seven Countries*...(See previous note for full reference)

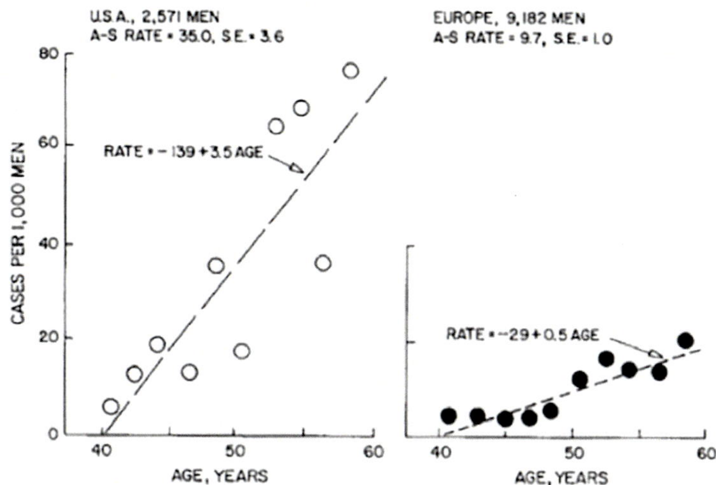

Figure 3.3 Age and the prevalence of old myocardial infarction among American railroad men and among men in the European cohorts. Cases per 1,000 men per two-year age class and the regression of the prevalence rate on age. A-S *rate* = rate per 1,000 men standardized by single years of age.

Figure 3.3 from *Seven Countries* (1980). Reprinted by permission of the publisher from *SEVEN COUNTRIES: A MULTIVARIATE ANALYSIS OF DEATH AND CORONARY HEART DISEASE* by Ancel Keys, p. 52, Cambridge, Mass.: Harvard University Press, Copyright © 1980 by the President and Fellows of Harvard College.

When participants were recruited for the Seven Countries Study some of the men recruited had already suffered a heart attack (called old myocardial infarction in the book). "But there were marked differences among the population samples. While CHD was recorded for 4.6 percent of the Americans and 3.6 percent for Finns, the prevalence of CHD was only 0.9 percent or less in nine of the other cohorts."[3] Ancel Keys graphed the number of cases with an old myocardial infarction per 1,000 men for each age class.[4] On the left side, the data for American men in the

3. Ibid., page 34.

Seven Countries Study were plotted, and on the right, the data for European men in the study were plotted. Quite unusual was the observation that American men had suffered previous myocardial infarctions at 3.6 times the rate that the Europeans had suffered them, and the rate increased faster with age in Americans, too.

Ancel Keys could not explain the large difference in the rates of coronary heart disease cases observed in the U.S. cohort pulled from the United States Railroad Study (35.0 per 1,000 men standardized by single years of age) compared to the European cohorts (9.7 per 1,000 men standardized by single years of age).

A major difference in these two populations was that the men in the U.S. cohort from the United States Railroad Study were all employed in fairly complex jobs, whereas the men in the European cohorts were largely from rural locations where farming was the predominant occupation. In the next chapter, I suggest an additional hypothesis that may partially explain the major difference observed in the basic coronary heart disease rates between the U.S. cohort and the combined European cohorts.

4. Ibid., page 52.

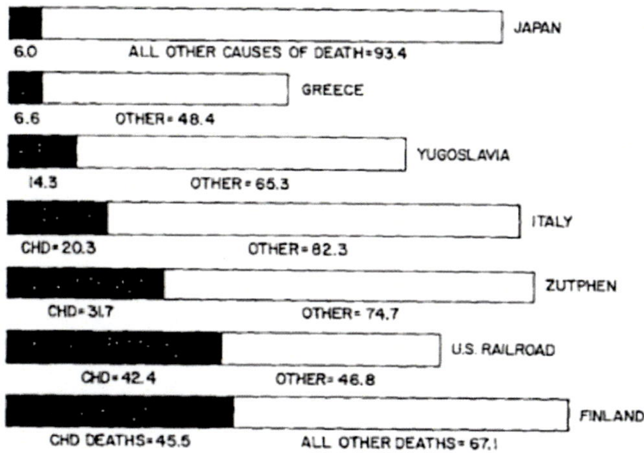

Figure 4.2. Ten-year age-standardized death rates per 10,000 from coronary heart disease and from all other causes, with the cohorts grouped by countries.

Figure 4.2 from *Seven Countries* (1980). Dark bars are coronary heart disease deaths and open bars are deaths from all other causes. Reprinted by permission of the publisher from *SEVEN COUNTRIES: A MULTIVARIATE ANALYSIS OF DEATH AND CORONARY HEART DISEASE* by Ancel Keys, p. 77, Cambridge, Mass.: Harvard University Press, Copyright © 1980 by the President and Fellows of Harvard College.

In figure 4.2 of Seven Countries, Dr. Keys graphed for each country the ten-year rates of death per 10,000 (age-adjusted) from coronary heart disease and also deaths from all other causes.[5]

Note that although the U.S. coronary heart disease death rate was higher than those for the other countries, except for Finland, the overall U.S. death rate was lower than that observed in four of the participating countries. This observation may reflect other aspects of American life such as availability of antibiotics, basic quality of the overall diet, and physical environment factors such as reliable transportation and sanitation.

5. Ibid., page 77.

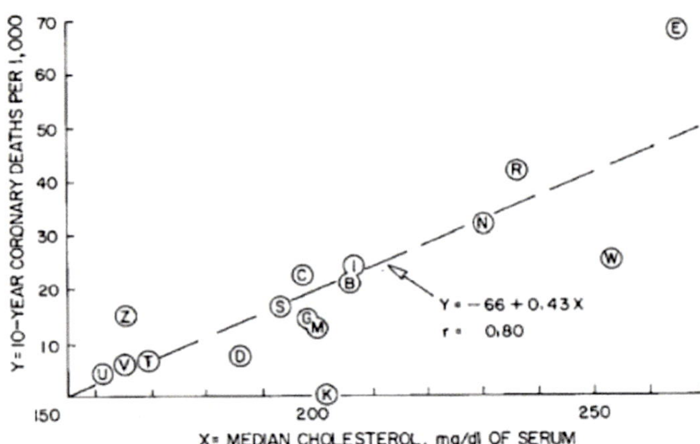

Figure 8.2. Coronary heart disease age-standardized ten-year death rates of the cohorts versus the median serum cholesterol levels (mg per dl) of the cohorts. All men judged free of coronary heart disease at entry. The coefficient of correlation is r = 0.82. Cohorts as in figure 8.1.

Figure 8.2 from *Seven Countries* (1980). The letters within circles designate a specific area or country. The cohorts are B = Belgrade; C = Crevalcore; D = Dalmatia; E = east Finland; G = Corfu; I = Italian railroad; K = Crete; M = Montegiorgio; N = Zutphen; R = American railroad; S = Slavonia; T = Tanushimaru; U = Ushibuka; V = Velika Krsna; W = west Finland; Z = Zrenjanin. All of the men graphed were free of coronary artery disease upon entry into the Seven Countries Study. Reprinted by permission of the publisher from *SEVEN COUNTRIES: A MULTIVARIATE ANALYSIS OF DEATH AND CORONARY HEART DISEASE* by Ancel Keys, p. 122, Cambridge, Mass.: Harvard University Press, Copyright © 1980 by the President and Fellows of Harvard College.

In Figure 8.2 the 10-year coronary death rate per 1,000 men (age-adjusted) of each cohort was graphed versus the medium serum cholesterol concentration (mg/dL) of that cohort.[6] This is one of the famous relationships from the study where coronary heart disease was highly associated with serum cholesterol levels across the various geographic areas studied. As will be described

6. Ibid., page 122.

later, this relationship is complicated by many factors. An interesting observation was that the rate of coronary heart disease in Crete (K) was zero even though the cohort's serum concentration of cholesterol was close to 200 mg/dL.

124 | Seven Countries

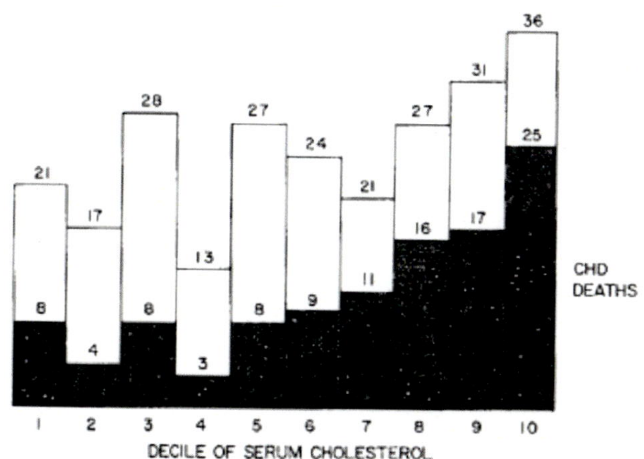

Figure 8.3. Numbers of ten-year deaths of American railroad men, free of coronary heart disease at entry, in the age- and cohort-specific decile classes of entry serum cholesterol level. Figures at the top of the shaded columns show numbers of deaths from coronary heart disease.

Figure 8.3 from *Seven Countries* (1980). Reprinted by permission of the publisher from *SEVEN COUNTRIES: A MULTIVARIATE ANALYSIS OF DEATH AND CORONARY HEART DISEASE* by Ancel Keys, p. 124, Cambridge, Mass.: Harvard University Press, Copyright © 1980 by the President and Fellows of Harvard College.

In figure 8.3 the total deaths (upper numbers) and the deaths from coronary heart disease (lower numbers above the shaded regions) from the American railroad men cohort were plotted according to the decile classes of serum cholesterol concentration upon entry into the study.[7] Deaths from coronary artery disease appeared to be associated with serum cholesterol concentration but not across the lower five decile classes. It appears that coronary heart disease was associated with serum cholesterol level only at high serum cholesterol concentrations. To quote Dr. Keys, "From the evidence it appears that the serum cholesterol concentration is an important risk factor for the incidence of coronary heart disease at levels of perhaps 220 mg/dl or more."[8] Dr. Keys was careful not to comment that there is a threshold concentration of cholesterol over which risk for coronary heart disease is increased. But at the time there was considerable debate whether there was in fact a threshold concentration for cholesterol in the blood.

Larger studies, performed after the Seven Countries Studies, showed that the relationship between coronary heart disease and serum cholesterol did not display a threshold type of response. This conclusion was made absolutely clear after analysis of the later MRFIT study, a massive study carried out in 18 cities and 22 clinical centers in the United States and funded by the National Heart, Lung, and Blood Institute of the National Institutes of Health.[9] The data published in 1986 from the Multiple Risk Factor Intervention Trial (MRFIT), which studied 356,222 men aged 35 to 57 years, showed that the relationship between serum cholesterol and coronary heart disease did not display a threshold, and that risk for coronary heart disease in middle-aged American men is "a continuously graded one." Coronary heart disease risk was found to be progressively higher with increased blood cholesterol concentration at every cholesterol level above 160 mg/dL. The results of the MRFIT study were confirmed through the entire follow-up period including in the 25-year

7. Ibid., page 124.
8. Ibid., page 135.
9. Stamler J, Wentworth D, Neaton JD (and the MRFIT Research Group). (1986) Is relationship between serum cholesterol and risk of premature death from coronary heart disease continuous and graded? *JAMA* 256(20): 2823-2828. http://jama.jamanetwork.com/article.aspx?articleid=363231

follow-up report.[10] The relationship between serum cholesterol and coronary heart disease held up when the results were "controlled for age, systolic blood pressure, number of cigarettes smoked per day, diabetes status, race and ethnicity, and study geographic site..."[11] The data in figure 8.3 of *Seven Countries* probably reflected its smaller cohort number and the short follow-up time (10 years) that was the only data available at the time *Seven Countries* was published in 1980.

10. Stamler J, Neaton JD. (2008) The Multiple Risk Factor Intervention Trial (MRFIT)—Importance Then and Now. *JAMA* 300(11):1343-1345. http://jama.jamanetwork.com/article.aspx?articleid=18255
11. Ibid., page 1343.

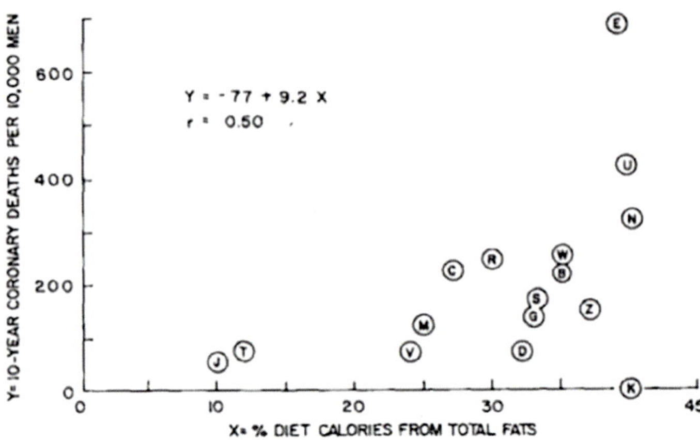

Figure 14.2. Ten-year coronary death rates of the cohorts plotted against the percentage of dietary calories supplied by total fats. Cohorts as in figure 14.1.

Figure 14.2 from *Seven Countries* (1980). The cohorts are B = Belgrade; C = Crevalcore; D = Dalmatia; E = east Finland; G = Corfu; J = Ushibuka; K = Crete; M = Montegiorgio; N = Zutphen; R = Rome railroad; S = Slavonia; T = Tanushimaru; U = American railroad; V = Velika Krsna; W = west Finland; Z = Zrenjanin. All of the men graphed were free of coronary artery disease upon entry into the Seven Countries Study. Reprinted by permission of the publisher from *SEVEN COUNTRIES: A MULTIVARIATE ANALYSIS OF DEATH AND CORONARY HEART DISEASE* by Ancel Keys, p. 251, Cambridge, Mass.: Harvard University Press, Copyright © 1980 by the President and Fellows of Harvard College.

In Figure 14.2 the 10-year coronary death rate (per 1,000 men, age-adjusted) of each cohort was graphed versus the mean percent of Kcal intake from total fat in the diet.[12] This is another famous relationship that emanated from the Seven Countries Study. If you draw a vertical dotted line at 40% of total Kcal from fat, east Finland, the United States, the Netherlands, and the island of Crete fall on that line. The data points along this line show that the effects of total dietary fat are complicated

12. Keys A. et al. (1980) Seven Countries...(full reference in chapter 1), page 251.

and modulated by other factors. The highest data point, East Finland, is interesting because this area did, indeed, have a very high intake of fat that was enriched in saturated fat from animal sources. The high number of deaths due to coronary heart disease in east Finland certainly fits Dr. Keys's hypothesis concerning saturated fat.

The data point for deaths in the U.S. cohort reflects the influence of diet and many other factors that were discussed earlier in this chapter. The data point that was most interesting was that from the Crete (marked with a K) cohort. Although men from Crete consumed a high fat diet (40% of total Kcal from fat), there were zero deaths from coronary heart disease. We now know that this low rate was the result of their consumption of the Mediterranean diet and the protective effects of a high intake of olive oil and marine fats that contain omega-3 fatty acids. These data illustrate the importance of the type of fat consumed in the diet. In *How to Eat Well and Stay Well the Mediterranean Way*, Dr. Keys and Margaret Keys wrote that this finding was instrumental in convincing them that the Mediterranean diet was protective against coronary heart disease.[13]

What were the final conclusions of the book, *Seven Countries*?

Dr. Keys's main conclusions, presented in the 1980 book, were (from page 341): "Our ten year finding, and concordance with other studies, make it clear that the big three risk factors for coronary heart disease now established are age, blood pressure, and serum cholesterol. The findings about cigarette smoking as a risk factor indicate that here, too, relationships are not as simple as first supposed."[14]

What happened in the United States after the results of

13. Keys A, Keys M. (1975) How to Eat Well and Stay Well the Mediterranean Way. Garden City, New York: Doubleday & Company.
14. Ibid., page 341.

the Seven Countries Study were published in the scientific literature?

After the early reports from Ancel Keys and other researchers, there was a concerted effort by certain government panels and private organizations, such as the American Heart Association, to advocate for lower dietary fat, especially saturated fat, in the American diet. In addition, steps were taken by doctors and medical organizations to develop better testing and treatment strategies for patients with CHD. Although the exact reasoning and outcomes have been debated, after the public responded to these recommendations, beneficial effects on health were eventually observed with about a 10- to 15-year delay. For example, in 1960, several studies measured the mean serum cholesterol concentration in adults at about 230 mg/dL in American adults.[15] The table that follows also shows how the serum cholesterol concentration increases with age. However, the decrease in serum cholesterol level observed in men 65-74 years old is historically attributed to the loss of men from the group because of deaths from coronary heart disease in the men with the highest serum cholesterol concentrations. The mean values observed in 1960 are very close to the values for total blood cholesterol that Ancel Keys measured in adult men in Minnesota in the 1950s.

15. Vital and Health Statistics, National Health Survey, Serum Cholesterol Levels in Adults, United States- 1960-1964, March 1963, Washington, D.C.

Serum Cholesterol in 1960

Table G. Mean serum cholesterol levels, by sex and age for specified populations

Sex and age	White				Negro	
	Total U.S. HES 1960-62	Framingham, Mass. 1958-60	Tecumseh, Mich. 1959-60	Evans County, Ga. 1960-62	South, HES 1960-62	Evans County, Ga. 1960-62
	Mean serum cholesterol in mg. per 100 ml.					
Men						
25-34 years	207	---	205	203	195	192
35-44 years	228	233	221	220	217	208
45-54 years	231	237	233	223	227	214
55-64 years	234	235	229	226	230	215
65-74 years	230	---	224	221	224	220
Women						
25-34 years	198	---	196	199	194	199
35-44 years	214	217	212	221	212	219
45-54 years	234	246	230	237	227	220
55-64 years	265	262	251	259	243	237
65-74 years	267	---	256	260	266	243

VITAL and HEALTH STATISTICS

Serum Cholesterol Levels of Adults

United States - 1960-1962

about

230 mg/dL on average

Screen shot of table of Vital and Health Statistics from the U.S. National Health Survey, published March 1963.

The concentrations of total blood cholesterol were measured in later years in the National Health and Nutrition Examination Surveys (NHANES). The data and their analysis from three of the NHANES studies were recently reported in 2010 by Cohen and colleagues.[16] The data displayed below is only a small portion of the data presented in Table 3 in the article by Cohen et al. This article contains a wealth of information concerning how blood

16. Cohen JD, Cziraky MJ, Cai Q, Wallace A, Wasser T, Crouse JR, Jacobson TA. (2010) 30-year trends in serum lipids among United States adults: results from the National Health and Nutrition Examination Surveys II, III, and 1999-2006. *Am J Cardiol* 106(7):969-75. http://www.ncbi.nlm.nih.gov/pubmed/20854959

lipids have changed over the past 30 to 40 years and an in depth discussion of the causes.

Mean total cholesterol levels (20 – 74 years) as reported by the NHANES studies 1976 to 2006 (Total cholesterol in mg/dL with (standard errors)).

Group:	Men	Women
NHANES II 1976-1980 (n=5,792)	209.3 (1.3)	209.6 (1.3)
NHANES III 1988-1994 (n=7,012)	203.4 (1.1)	203.2 (1.3)
NHANES 1999-2006 (n=8,174)	199.5 (1.1)	200.9 (0.8)

By 1976, the mean blood cholesterol concentration in American adults had fallen to about 209 mg/dL in both men and women. The NHANES III (1988-1994) study noted a further reduction in blood total cholesterol down to 203 mg/dL for both men and women. By the 1999 to 2006 period total cholesterol concentrations had fallen to approximately 200 mg/dL. It should be noted that statin drugs were first introduced in 1987, so that the drop in total cholesterol concentrations through NHANES III was not due to the effects of this drug. The decline in total blood cholesterol from 1994 to 2006 most likely included effects due to statins and other drugs. Needless-to-say, the drop in the mean cholesterol from 1960 to 2006 was sufficient to have a positive outcome on cardiovascular diseases. During this time, the number of heart attacks peaked at about 1950 and started to progressively fall afterwards (see data from the American Heart Association below).

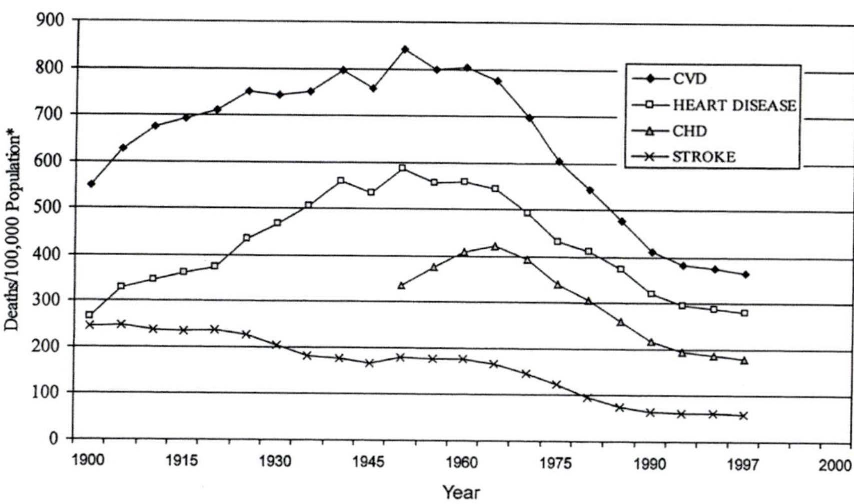

Cooper R. et al. (2000) Trends and disparities in coronary heart disease... Circulation 102(25): 3137-3147.

Although there was a lag period of 5-10 years after the major results concerning diet and blood cholesterol and coronary heart disease were announced, the epidemic of deaths from coronary heart disease started to decrease starting about 1965.[17] Again, there may be other factors (i.e., better treatments for high blood pressure, lower smoking rates) involved in this turnaround, but the decline in serum cholesterol concentrations is considered a powerful contributor.

The overall results were such that many men who would have died in their 40s and 50s of heart attacks died much later, in their 70s and 80s. My father had his first attack at the age of 85. Many of us have benefited greatly by having our fathers live 20-30

17. Cooper R, Cutler J, Desvigne-Nickens P, Fortmann SP, Friedman L, Havlik R, Hogelin G, Marler J, McGovern P, Morosco G, Mosca L, Pearson T, Stamler J, Stryer D, Thom T. (2000) Trends and disparities in coronary heart disease, stroke, and other cardiovascular diseases in the United States: findings of the national conference on cardiovascular disease prevention. *Circulation* 102(25): 3137-3147. http://circ.ahajournals.org/content/102/25/3137.long

years longer because Ancel Keys and his colleagues advanced and studied the diet/cholesterol/coronary heart disease hypothesis.

Next Chapter: The insidious factor that increased coronary heart disease in the United States in the 1950s that was unknown until the late 1980s.

5.

THE "SOMETHING ELSE HYPOTHESIS" - A INSIDIOUS CAUSE OF INCREASED CORONARY HEART DISEASE IN THE U.S. IN THE 1950S

The findings in the 1950s and 1960s that high blood cholesterol was associated with coronary heart disease and that dietary saturated fat and, to a much lesser extent, dietary cholesterol, could influence blood cholesterol levels, initiated a three to four decades war on the intake of fat as a causative factor of cardiovascular disease. The crucial problem with this approach was the fact that the real story was much more complicated than any investigator could have imagined at the time.

There was one additional factor that needs to be discussed here that was (and is) almost never taken into account in a review of the development of the "fat as evil" story. This insidious factor may have inserted a major confounding effect into the entire story of fat as the cause of cardiovascular disease.

In the 1700s chemists learned how to convert liquid whale oils and other fats into a hard substance so that candles could be made. This process involved sequential boiling. Later on, chemists devised a simple process to harden vegetable oils. This involved pumping hydrogen gas into oils so that unsaturated fatty acids became saturated fatty acids. In the 1940s after World War II, American food companies supported the introduction of large amounts of this product onto the foodscape in order to find a way to sell excess liquid vegetable oils. The product was called margarine and it was advertised to be healthy compared to "unhealthy" butter, and it was cheaper, too.[1] In this searing account of the entire history of margarine and the politics involved, Dr. Schleifer describes how the Center for Science in the Public Interest (CSPI) supported the use of hydrogenated oils even as late as 1993, "From 1981 to 1993 CSPI routinely endorsed trans fats as a healthier alternative to saturated fats, although in doing so its tone was often defensive, perhaps because a few scientists were already suggesting associations between trans fats and disease. But CSPI's endorsement of trans fats during the 1980s was largely consistent with most contemporaneous scientific authorities, including the National Research Council and the Institute of Medicine."[2] There was a major problem with margarine, unknown at the time: during the process of hardening of liquid vegetable oil into solid bars, toxic fatty acids, called trans fatty acids, were formed during the hydrogenation process. The devastating effects of trans fats on blood lipids were first published in 1990.[3] This article by Mensink and Katan, and their

1. Schleifer D. (2012) The Perfect Solution: How Trans Fats Became the Healthy Replacement for Saturated Fats. *Technology and Culture* 53(1): 94-119. http://muse.jhu.edu/login?auth=0&type=summary&url=/journals/technology_and_culture/v053/53.1.schleifer.html
2. Ibid., page 110.
3. Mensink R, Katan M. (1990) Effect of Dietary Trans Fatty Acids on High-

subsequent publications, sent shock waves throughout the food and nutrition communities. As quoted by Dr. Schleifer[4] and reported originally in the *New York Times*, influential epidemiologist Walter Willett, chairman of the Department of Nutrition at the Harvard School of Public Health, stated, "There was a lot of resistance from the scientific community because a lot of people had made their careers telling people to eat margarine instead of butter. . . . When I was a physician in the 1980s, that's what I was telling people to do and unfortunately we were often sending them to their graves prematurely."[5] This quote demonstrates how truly unknown the toxic effects of trans fatty acids were among nutritionists and clinicians in the period before the reports of Katan. As will be discussed later, even Dr. Keys was unaware of the effects of trans fats at this time.

On the slide below the per capita consumption of margarine is shown for the U.S.[6] Note that the half maximal consumption of margarine occurred in the United States about 1953, and that intake leveled off about 1969 and lasted as a long plateau until 1990.

Density and Low-Density Lipoprotein Cholesterol in Healthy Subjects. *N Eng J Med.* 323: 439-445. http://www.nejm.org/doi/full/10.1056/NEJM199008163230703

4. Ibid., page 118.
5. Kim Severson and Melanie Warner. (2005) "Fat Substitute Is Pushed Out of the Kitchen," *New York Times*, 13 February, A1, http://www.nytimes.com/2005/02/13/business/13transfat.html
6. Brian Gould, Agricultural and Applied Economics, UW Madison, http://future.aae.wisc.edu/data/annual_values/by_area/2213?period=complete&tab=sales (Downloaded 3-22-2014)

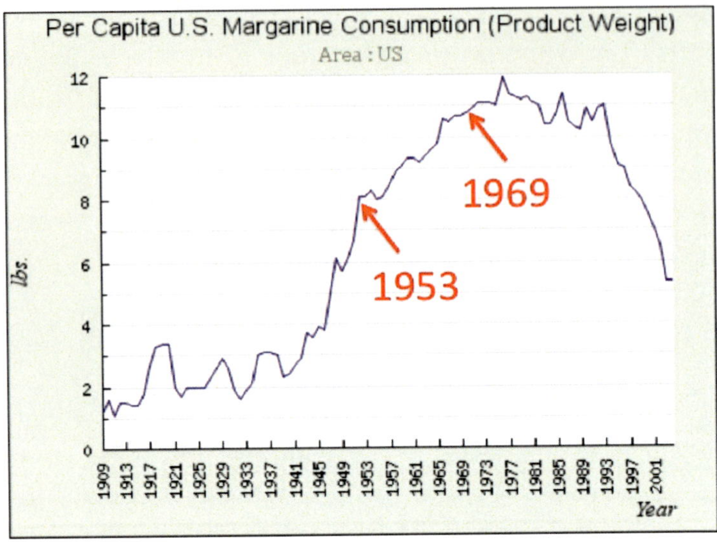

© Brian Gould, *Agricultural and Applied Economics*, UW Madison
http://future.aae.wisc.edu/data/annual_values/by_area/2213?period=complete&tab=sales
Downloaded 3-22-2014

Margarine consumption (in pounds/year) in the United States, from Dr. Brian Gould.

In the figures below Blasbalg and colleagues[7] charted how the use of fats and oils changed in the U.S. during the 20th century. The first figure shows how butter usage decreased during the 1930s to the 1970s and was replaced by margarine and shortening. Lard use also decreased in the middle part of the century.

7. Blasbalg TL, Hibbeln JR, Ramsden CE, Majchrzak SF, Rawlings RR. (2011) Changes in consumption of omega-3 and omega-6 fatty acids in the United States during the 20th century. *Am J Clin Nutr* 93(5): 950-962. http://ajcn.nutrition.org/content/93/5/950.long

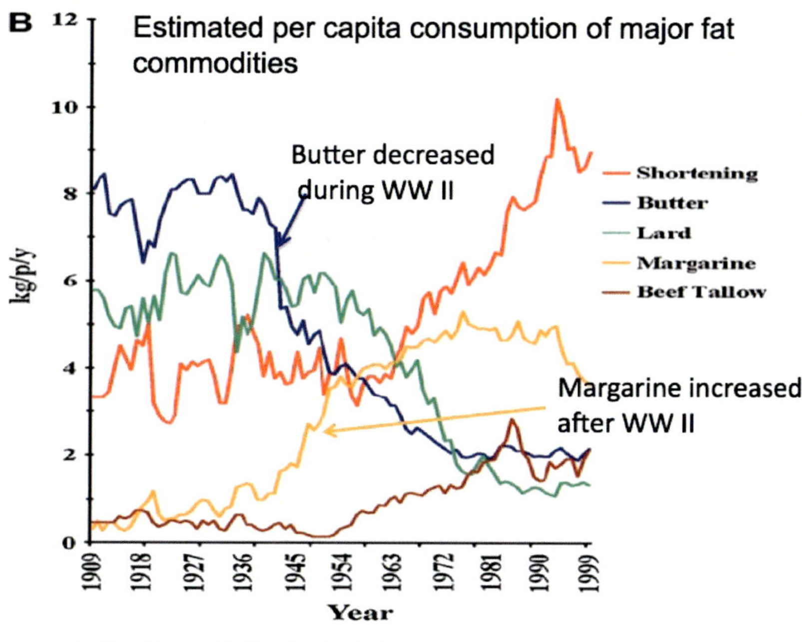

Panel B from figure 1 of Blasbalg *et al.* (2011).

The next figure charts the use of vegetable oils through the century. Starting in the late 1950s and 1960s the use of soybean oil skyrocketed. In the late 1980s, canola oil, developed in Canada to replace palm oil imported from Southeast Asia, appeared on the U.S. market, and due to aggressive advertising, its use increased rapidly over the next 10 years. Note that olive oil usage remained fairly low and consistent over the entire period. The rather late increase in the use of soybean oil (starting about 1965) suggests it could not have been involved in the post World War II increase in coronary heart disease, but the timing does raise the possibility that it may have had partial effects concerning the decrease in the rates of coronary heart disease later in the 1900s.

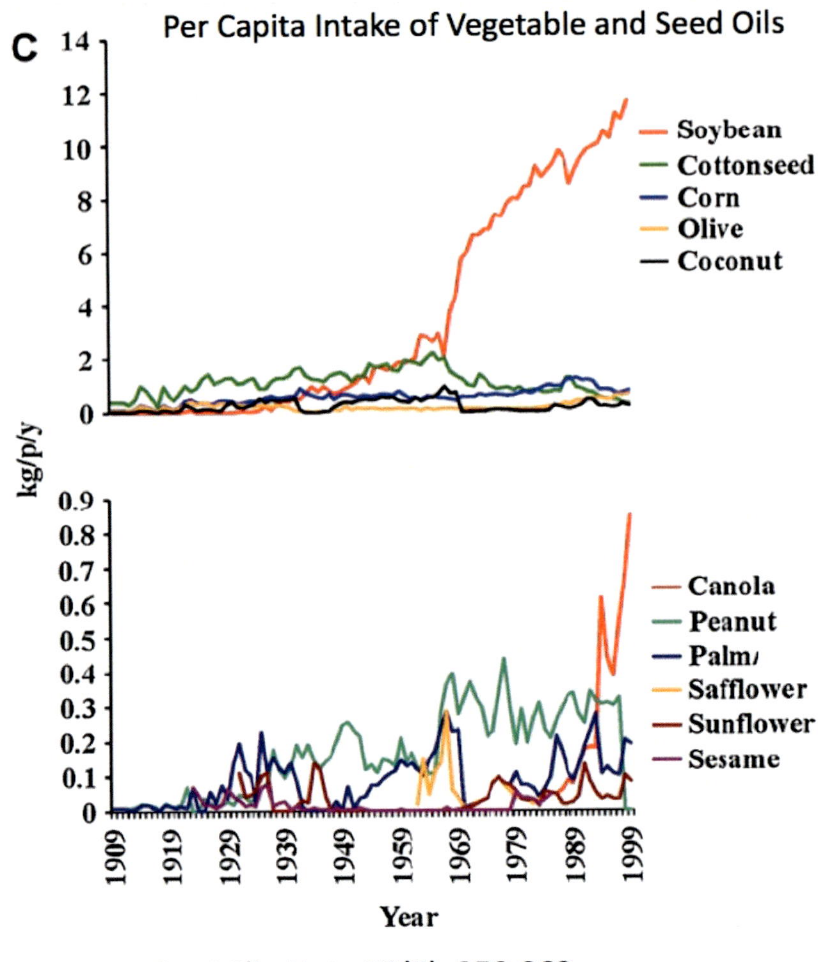

Panel C from figure 1 of Blasbalg *et al.* (2011).

The next figure shows the composition of margarine versus butter and tub (soft) margarine.[8]

8. Zock PL, Katan MB. (1997) Butter, margarine and serum lipoproteins. *Atherosclerosis* 131(1):7-16. http://www.ncbi.nlm.nih.gov/pubmed/9180239

Types of Fatty Acids in Butter and Margarine

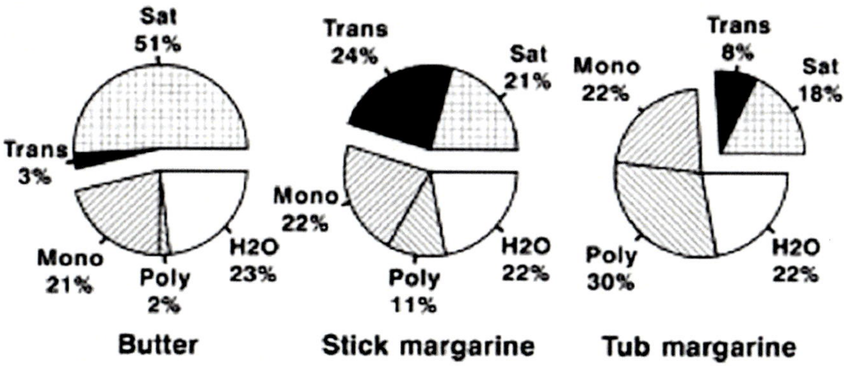

Figure 1 from Peter L Zock, Martijn B Katan (1997) Atherosclerosis 131(1): 7-16. See extended legend from this figure in the text.

The extended legend for this figure was:

> Composition, in grams per 100 grams of product, of butter and of the average stick margarines (*N*=32) and tub margarines (*N*=17) used in the 20 experiments reviewed. Sat, saturated fatty acids; Trans, *trans* fatty acids; Mono, *cist*-monounsaturated fatty acids; Poly, polyunsaturated fatty acids; and H20, water plus glycerol and other minor substances. Butter contains about 220 mg, vegetable margarines less than 1 mg, and margarines made with animal fats 70–275 mg cholesterol per 100 grams of product.

Whereas butter is 51% saturated and contains 3% trans fatty acids, margarine contains 21% saturated and 24% trans fatty acids. The 24% trans is considered much more dangerous and unhealthy than the saturated fatty acids found in butter. Studies have shown that trans fatty acids both raise serum low density lipoprotein (LDL) cholesterol and lower high density lipoprotein (HDL) cholesterol, changes that would double the negative effects and, therefore, greatly increase the risk for coronary heart disease.[9] The composition of stick margarine was undoubtedly more atherogenic than the composition of butter. Therefore, increasing consumption of margarine would probably counter act much of the improvements in coronary heart disease risk accomplished by lowering total intake of fat and cholesterol in the American diet during the period from the 1950s to the 1990s.

The above figures paint a complicated picture concerning the role of changes in general fat intake on the increase in coronary heart disease in the early to mid 1900s. It is difficult to assign blame for increased cardiovascular disease to general changes in fat consumption during this period. However, the insidious and dangerous biochemical effects discovered for margarine by Mensink and Katan[10] point a very interesting finger at this highly toxic margarine food product. One interesting historical note is that Drs. Ancel Keys and Martijn Katan were on very cordial terms, and there are several letters in the Ancel Keys archives that show that Dr. Katan kept Dr. Keys informed of his studies on the health effects of trans fats.[11]

9. Ibid., page 7.
10. Mensink R, Katan M. (1990) Effect of Dietary Trans Fatty Acids on High-Density and Low-Density Lipoprotein Cholesterol in Healthy Subjects. *N Eng J Med.* 323: 439-445. http://www.nejm.org/doi/full/10.1056/NEJM199008163230703
11. Letter, dated July 10, 1989, from Dr. Katan to Dr. Keys, where Dr. Katan thanked Dr. Keys for his letter dated June 12, 1989. Dr. Katan had previously sent Dr. Keys two of his articles. In the July 10th letter, Dr. Katan wrote, "I am glad you found some merit in it." Archives of Dr. Ancel Keys and the Seven Countries Study. Division of Epidemiology and Community Health, School of Public Health, Univ. of Minnesota, 1300 S. Second St. WBOB Suite 300, Minneapolis, MN 55454. Courtesy of Dr. Henry Blackburn. http://www.epi.umn.edu/cvdepi/

Studies in Finland, the Country with the Highest Rate of Coronary Heart Disease in the World

In the Seven Countries Study, the country (actually an area of that country) that had the highest incidence of coronary heart disease was eastern Finland. The population of eastern Finland was known to have a very high intake of fat, including a very high use of butter in everyday meals (see Ancel Keys's comments on this in chapter 2). Therefore, if high intakes of saturated fat and cholesterol were responsible for the high rates of coronary heart disease, then efforts to decrease their intake in eastern Finland would have the best chance to show the efficacy of lowering serum cholesterol. An added factor that would make eastern Finland an appropriate place to observe this is that through most of this period, margarine intake was fairly low and constant. Therefore, if the people of Finland decreased their serum cholesterol concentrations through diet, especially those with very high cholesterol levels, the full beneficial effects of lipid lowering on coronary heart disease should have been observed directly. This is exactly what happened. Health officials instituted programs to educate the population on the effects of eating high levels of fat, and their intake of saturated fat did indeed fall.[12]

The figure below shows the decreased intake of table fats in Finland.[13] During the course of the study the intake of total table fats, and butter in particular, decreased. The consumption of margarine stayed consistently low. Interestingly, the consumption of cheese, not considered a table fat, increased during the study.

12. Pietinen P, Vartiainen E, Seppänen R, Aro A, Puska P. (1996) Changes in diet in Finland from 1972 to 1992: impact on coronary heart disease risk. *Preventive Medicine* 25(3): 243-250. http://www.sciencedirect.com/science/article/pii/S0091743596900535
13. Ibid., page 247.

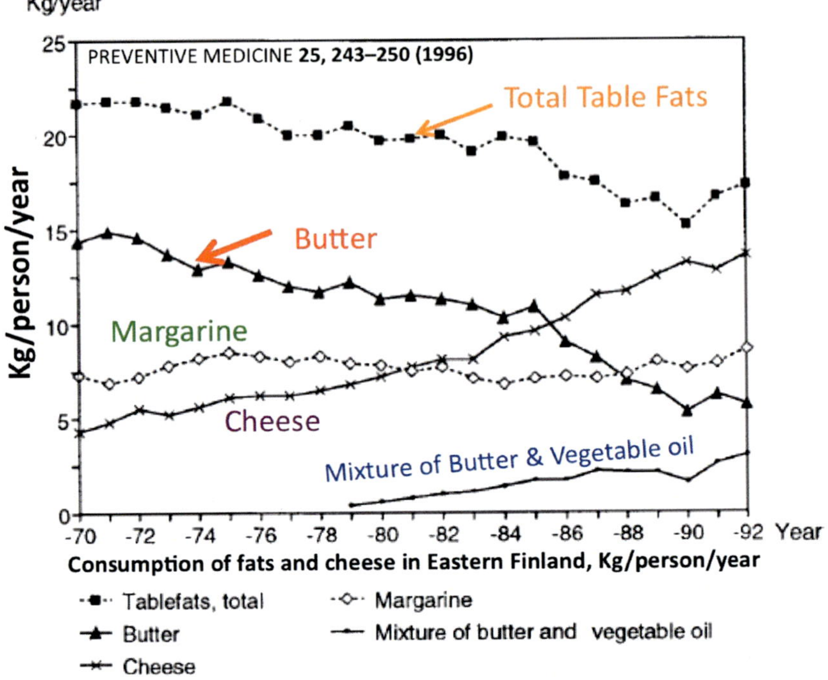

Figure 4 from Pietinen *et al.* (1996) *Prev Medicine* 25(3): 235-250. Arrows and labels added by the author.

Below is a figure that shows serum cholesterol distribution in men, 30 to 59 years, in Finland by study year.[14] From 1972 to 1992, the distribution of cholesterol shifted left, such that the mean cholesterol in men decreased from 262 mg/dL to 228 mg/dL. In a 25-year period from about 1970 to 1995, mortality from coronary heart disease in eastern Finland decreased to about less than half of that originally observed, with decreased cholesterol concentrations determined to be statistically

14. Jousilahti P, Vartiainen E, Pekkanen J, Tuomilehto J, Sundvall J, Puska P. (1998) Serum cholesterol distribution and coronary heart disease risk: observations and predictions among middle-aged population in eastern Finland. *Circulation* 97(11): 1087-1094. http://circ.ahajournals.org/content/97/11/1087.long

responsible for about half of the decrease in coronary heart disease (the other half being explained statistically by lowered smoking and decreased blood pressure).

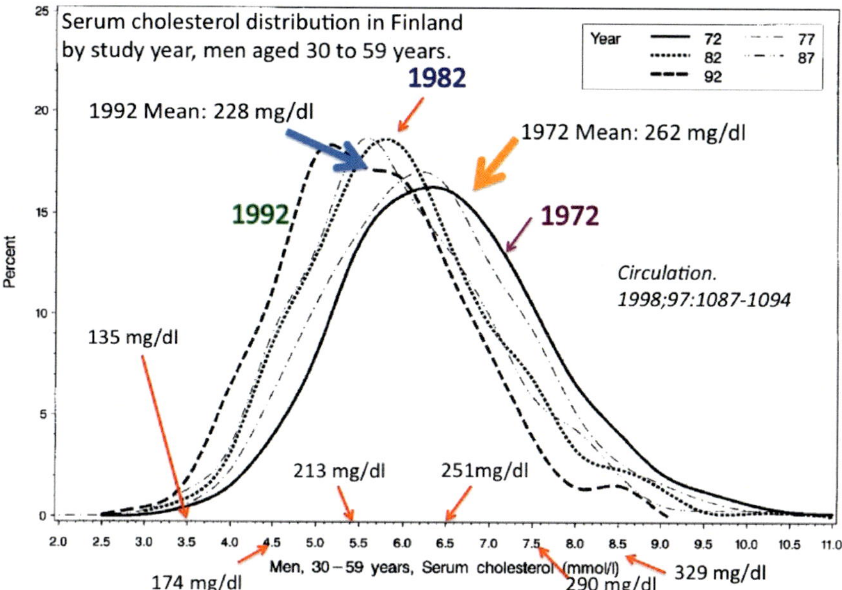

Figure 1 from Jousilahti *et al.* (1998) *Circulation* 97: 1087-1094. Arrows and descriptors added by the author. The graph shows the distribution of cholesterol concentrations improved in Finland from 1972 to 1992. In places I have indicated the cholesterol concentrations in mg/dl, the unit used in the U.S.

In Finland, the serum cholesterol concentrations decreased steadily from about 1970 onward, and the incidence of coronary heart disease also decreased during the period.

The long-term results of the intervention in Finland, called the North Karelia Project, are described below.[15]

15. Oppenheimer GM, Blackburn H, Puska, P. (2011) From Framingham to North Karelia to U.S. Community-Based prevention programs: negotiating research

Smoking changed from 52% in men and 10% in women in 1972, to 32% in men and 17% in women in 1992, to 31% in men and 18% in women in 2007. Serum cholesterol (mmol/L) changed from 6.9 in men and 6.8 in women in 1972, to 5.9 in men and 5.6 in women in 1992, to 5.4 in men and 5.2 in women in 2007. Blood pressure (mmHg) changed from 149/92 in men and 153/92 in women in 1972, to 142/85 in men and 135/80 in women in 1992, to 138/83 in men and 134/78 in women in 2007. Coronary heart disease (mortality per 100,000 population) in males (ages 35 to 64 years) in North Karelia changed from 700 in 1970 to 300 in 1992 to 100 in 2007.

Two important quotes from this article are:

> As a result of the improved adult mortality rates, the estimated life expectancy at birth in Finland rose from 66.4/74.6 years (males/females) in 1971 to 75.8/82.8 years in 2006...[16]
>
> Separate analyses have shown that the observed reductions in population risk factor levels can account for most of the decline in coronary heart disease mortality. Of the single risk factors, reduction in serum cholesterol level had the greatest apparent impact.[17]

In the United States, the rate of deaths from coronary heart disease declined much slower, as did the serum cholesterol concentrations. As discussed earlier in this chapter, increased consumption of stick margarine, starting in the 1950s, may have been responsible for the lackluster U.S. response.

However, there is really no way of knowing how detrimental the increased consumption of margarine was for the American public. One thing is for sure, Dr. Ancel Keys had no idea that, exactly when his study was being conducted, the intake of a dangerous fat

agenda for coronary heart disease in the second half of the 20th Century. *Public Health Reviews* 33(2): 450-483. http://www.publichealthreviews.eu/show/i/10

16. Ibid., page 474.
17. Ibid., page 474.

(trans fat) was steadily increasing in the United States. This is the perfect example of the "Something Else Hypothesis," which posits that, in certain instances, something totally different, essentially an unknown unknown, may be the actual cause of the results being observed in a research study, and not the reasons the researchers have carefully extracted from analysis of the basic data. There was no way that Ancel Keys could have known that his entire study, at least the American portion of it, was affected by the introduction of margarine into the U.S. diet.

6.

THE KEYSES IN THE LAB; CONTRIBUTION TO THE DISCOVERY OF LDL

During the early period (1950-1955), when Ancel Keys was first traveling around the globe to collect data on cultural differences in diet, serum cholesterol level, and the prevalence of coronary heart disease (CHD), in order to determine what was responsible for different rates of CHD in different countries, he directed his laboratory at the University of Minnesota to develop biochemical markers for the upcoming epidemiology studies.[1] One of the methods that his laboratory became expert in was the measurement of blood cholesterol concentration and the separation of the alpha (now called high density lipoprotein

1. Anderson JT, Keys A, with the collaboration of Fidanza F, Keys, MH, Bronte-Stewart B, Kupcs P, and Werner L. (1956) Cholesterol in serum and lipoprotein fractions its measurement and stability. *Clinical Chemistry* 2(3): 145-159. http://www.clinchem.org/content/2/3/145.long

(HDL)) and beta (now called low density lipoprotein (LDL)) lipoprotein fractions from serum.

The Discovery of Low Density Lipoprotein (LDL) (See chapter 11 for an in-depth description of LDL)

When the number of heart attacks increased in several populations after World War II, research groups in several universities and clinics launched studies into the mystery of this disease. In a very short period of time in the late 1940s and early 1950s, several laboratories made discoveries that helped point to blood cholesterol as a possible factor. Often in scientific research, a paradigm-altering discovery is not made all at once by one person or laboratory, but is actually the sum of several smaller discoveries that, when added together, explain a biological or physical phenomenon in a new and revealing way. This is exactly what happened in the area of blood cholesterol and the discovery of LDL.

Let's briefly review the studies performed in the late 1940s and early 1950s that, when considered as an aggregate, can be labeled as the discovery of the lipoprotein, LDL. Some early observations pointed to the fact that cholesterol was not free in solution in blood, but existed in combination with proteins in the aqueous portion of blood called plasma or serum. Several methods were used to show this, including electrophoresis and ultracentrifugation.

In the 1940s, JL Oncley and EJ Cohn and colleagues at Harvard, using a combination of precipitation and ultracentrifugation methods, isolated beta-lipoprotein from human plasma and characterized its protein and lipid composition.[2] Their analysis for lipids and protein turned out to be very close to what we now accept as the composition of beta-lipoprotein (LDL).[3 4]

2. Oncley JL, Scatchard G, Brown A. (1947) Physical-chemical characteristics of certain of the proteins of normal human plasma. *J Phys Colloid Chem* (Jan). 51(1): 184-198. http://pubs.acs.org/doi/pdf/10.1021/j150451a014

The beta-lipoprotein (LDL) particle was determined to be 23% protein, 29% cholesteryl ester, 8% free cholesterol, 29% phospholipid, and 8% other esters (including triglyceride).[5] They also found that about 75% of the total blood cholesterol is in the beta-lipoprotein (LDL) fraction.[6] The following quote from these authors shows them to be ahead of their time in their understanding of the physiology of beta-lipoprotein (LDL):[7]

> This description of the composition and properties of the Beta-lipoprotein of human plasma is in keeping with the concept of its function as a carrier for certain lipids. By linkage with the polypeptide in the form of Beta-lipoprotein these lipids are rendered water-soluble and are freely transported in the blood stream without introducing any structure of radically different physical properties from those of the rest of the plasma proteins,...(it) is not a transport form for fat on its way to and from the fat depots, but rather is a specialized carrier molecule elaborated by the liver. The role of the Beta-lipoprotein as a carrier for vitamins and hormones is implied by the presence of carotenoids and estrogens in some of the molecules (Table III).

Working at the University of California-Berkeley, John Gofman's group also developed the method of centrifuging plasma or serum at high speed in the ultracentrifuge to obtain lipoproteins.[8]

With the development of this method, Gofman and colleagues,

3. Gurd FRN, Oncley JL, Edsall JT, Cohn EJ, (1949) The lipo-proteins of human plasma. *Discussions Faraday Society* 6: 70-74. http://pubs.rsc.org/en/Content/ArticleLanding/1949/DF/df9490600070#!divAbstract
4. Oncley JL, Gurd FRN, Melin M. (1950) Preparation and properties of serum and plasma proteins. XXV. Composition and properties of human serum beta-lipoprotein. *J Am Chem Society* 72: 458-464. http://pubs.acs.org/doi/abs/10.1021/ja01157a121
5. Ibid., page 460, Table II.
6. Ibid., page 463.
7. Ibid., page 464.
8. Gofman JW, Lindgren FT, and Elliott H. (1949) Ultracentrifugal studies lipoproteins of human serum. *J Biol Chem* 179: 973-979. http://www.jbc.org/content/179/2/973.full.pdf+html?sid=5e1a2fad-b3dc-411e-88e7-17a9962c6447

in an article published in *Science* in February 1950[9] reported that when rabbits were fed cholesterol, those that developed the most severe atherosclerosis contained an interesting lipoprotein particle in their plasma. His research group also observed that some humans contained a similar sized lipoprotein. This lipoprotein particle, now known as intermediate density lipoprotein (IDL), and also called pre-LDL by some, was about double the size of the main beta-lipoprotein (LDL) in human plasma. Gofman's group also observed, "The incidence of measurable concentrations of molecules of the...(intermediate density lipoprotein-author's insertion)...class is significantly higher in males from 20 to 40 years of age than in females of the same age group."[10]

In an article published in *Circulation* in August 1950,[11] Gofman's research group went on to observe that there was an increase in the intermediate density lipoprotein class in patients with coronary heart disease. When humans were fed low fat and cholesterol diets, these particles decreased greatly–in some subjects dropping almost to zero. Therefore, John Gofman linked lipoprotein particles, especially the class now known as intermediate density lipoprotein, with diseased states and with the diet. He later went on to publish many articles on lipoproteins and health. Quite interestingly, the atherogenic nature of intermediate density lipoproteins is still debated today.

In 1951 Howard Eder's group at the Cornell Medical Center in New York published two lengthy studies in the *American Journal of Medicine*[12] that utilized the laborious Cohn precipitation method to characterize different protein-lipid fractions in human serum.

9. Gofman JW, Lindgren, F, Elliott H, Mantz W, Hewitt J, Strisower B, Herring V, Lyon TP. (1950) The Role of Lipids and Lipoproteins in Atherosclerosis. *Science* 111: 166-171 and page 186.
10. Ibid., page 170.
11. Gofman JW, Jones HB, Lindgren FT, Lyon TP, Elliott HA, and Strisower B. (1950) Blood lipids and human atherosclerosis. *Circulation* 2:161-172.
12. Russ EM, Eder HA, Barr DP. (1951) Protein-lipid relationships in human plasma. I. In normal individuals. *Am J Med* (4): 468-479; Barr D P, Russ

They provided data from many patients and showed that the percentage of total cholesterol was increased in the beta-lipoprotein (LDL) fraction in patients with coronary heart disease.

However, in their second article, the most impressive finding was the decrease in cholesterol level in the alpha lipoprotein (HDL) fraction of blood in patients that were inflicted with a wide variety of disease states. Somehow, these extraordinary observations on the alpha fraction from Eder's lab were relegated to a lower importance in the medical community, and the importance of HDL in coronary heart disease was only revived in 1977 in the studies performed as part of the Framingham Study (see chapter 12).

In 1952 Swahn improved paper electrophoresis of plasma by providing a method to measure the lipids in each of the protein fractions.[13] In 1955 Oliver and Boyd used Swahn's method to measure the distribution of cholesterol between beta and alpha lipoproteins in the blood of patients with CHD.[14] Oliver and Boyd observed that the percentage of cholesterol in beta lipoproteins (LDL) was 72% in the control group versus 91% in the group with CHD, a result that was highly significant.

Contributions of Ancel and Margaret Keys to the Role of LDL in Atherosclerosis

In 1955, Dr. Keys and his colleagues published a very interesting and historically important article in the journal *Lancet* that gave insights into the role of LDL in the development of CHD.[15]

EM, Eder HA. (1951) Protein-lipid relationships in human plasma. II. In atherosclerosis and related conditions. *Am J Med* (4): 480-493.

13. Swahn B. (1952) A method for localization and determination of serum lipids after electrophoretical separation on filter paper. *Scand J Clin Lab Invest* 4, 98-103.
14. Oliver MF, Boyd GS. (1955) Serum lipoprotein patterns in coronary sclerosis and associated conditions. *Br Heart J.* 17(3):299-302. http://heart.bmj.com/content/17/3/299.long
15. Bronte-Stewart B, Keys A, Brock JF, with the collaboration of Moodie AD, Keys MH, Antonis A. (1955) Serum-Cholesterol, Diet, and Coronary Heart-

Ancel and Margaret Keys were invited to visit South Africa to work with Dr. J.F. Block, a well known physician and professor of medicine at the University of Cape Town. Together they designed a study to investigate the interrelationship of diet and blood cholesterol in three distinct populations in South Africa: the Bantus, who did not suffer from CHD; a group called "Cape Coloured," who consisted of immigrants from several Asian countries (primarily from India, Pakistan, and Malaysia); and a group who were descendents of several groups of Europeans who migrated to South Africa beginning with the Dutch in the mid-1600s. The Europeans, but not the other groups, suffered from high rates of CHD. Very important, all of the men recruited for this study were free of any signs of coronary heart disease and were healthy upon physical examination. Quite interestingly, Margaret Keys set up a temporary laboratory and was the technician who performed the cholesterol assays on the blood from all the men of these groups.

What the Keyses and their South African colleagues found was that total blood cholesterol concentration increased from a low of 166 in the Bantu, to 204 in the Cape Coloured (immigrants from Asia), to 234 in the group with European ancestry. The increase in total blood cholesterol appeared to correlate with the intake of animal fat in the diet. But the Keyses went further, and used the new electrophoresis method of Swahn to measure lipids in the alpha and beta fractions of blood. In their publication Keys and colleagues showed that when cholesterol increased in blood, the increase occurred primarily in the beta fraction (i.e., LDL).

Unlike the previous studies performed by the other research groups, this study was not performed in patients who had presented with severe disease. Keys's group made the distinct discovery that, in healthy populations, an increase in the consumption of animal fat was associated with an increase in

Disease, An Inter-racial Survey in the Cape Peninsula. *Lancet*, Nov 26 1955, 1103-1108 http://www.ncbi.nlm.nih.gov/pubmed/?term=13272336

blood cholesterol in the beta fraction, later called LDL. Therefore, since all the participants were healthy, the disease state of the patient was not the cause of the increased blood LDL cholesterol in their study. Quite interestingly, the increase was not related to total fat intake, but tracked with the intake of animal fat. The observations reported in their article were the first to show that LDL cholesterol was influenced by diet (primarily animal fat), and that high concentrations of LDL were not the result of some other condition that was associated with an illness or advanced disease state.

The South African study was the capstone of the series of studies that were performed by a number of research groups in the early 1950s that investigated the role of blood cholesterol in coronary heart disease. These studies culminated in the finding that a special protein-lipid particle in blood (first called beta particle but later called LDL) was closely associated with CHD, and that the concentration of LDL could be greatly affected by diet. Certainly, Dr. Ancel Keys and Margaret Keys were intrinsic contributors to the momentous scientific discovery of LDL. Later in this book, I will discuss the role of Margaret Keys in this momentous discovery, as she played an incredibly important role because she was the technician who, onsite in South Africa, measured the cholesterol concentrations in the participants' blood and performed the separation of the lipoprotein particles by paper electrophoresis. Below is a picture of Margaret Keys as she worked in the lab in South Africa.[16]

16. Picture of Margaret Keys during studies performed in South Africa. Archives of Dr. Ancel Keys and Margaret Keys, and the Seven Countries Study. Division of Epidemiology and Community Health, School of Public Health, Univ. of Minnesota, 1300 S. Second St. WBOB Suite 300, Minneapolis, MN 55454. Courtesy of Dr. Henry Blackburn. http://www.epi.umn.edu/cvdepi/

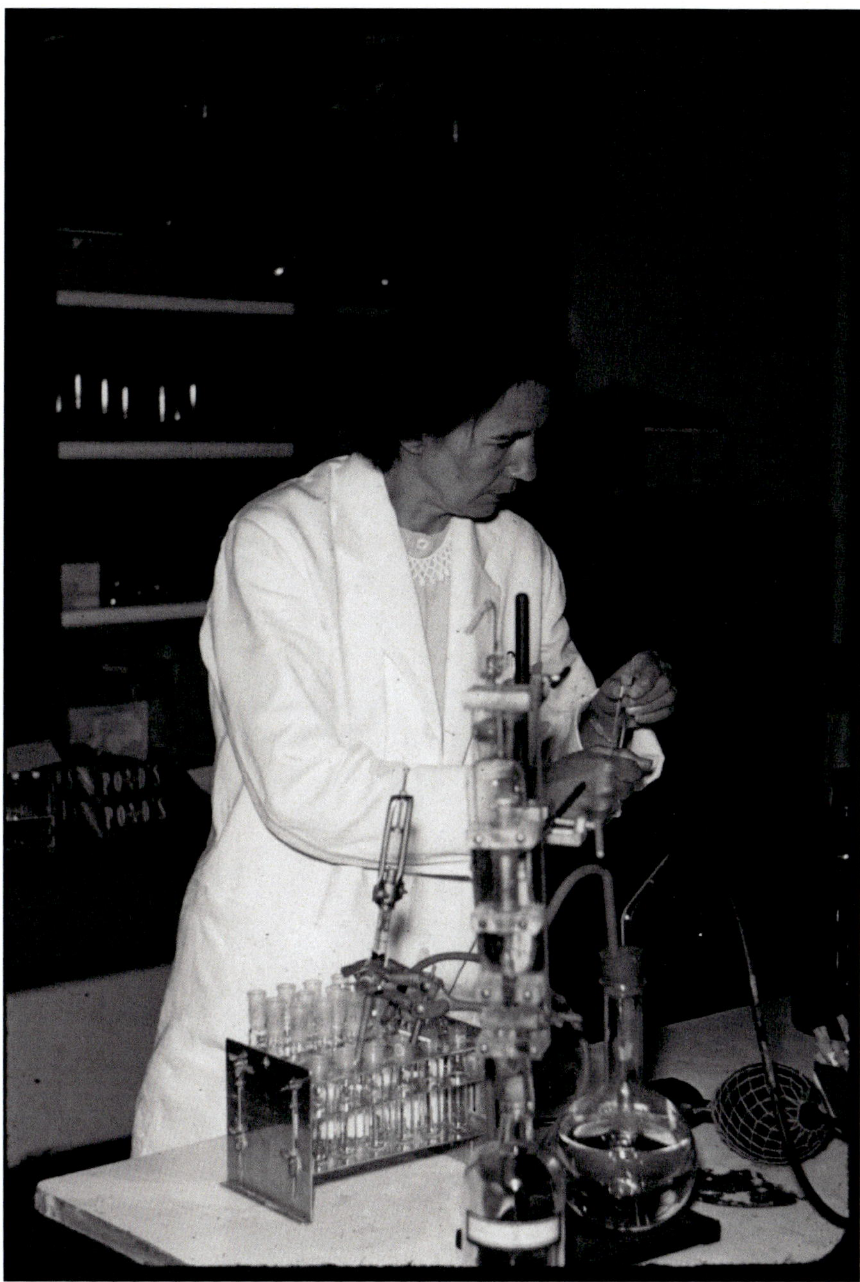

Margaret Keys working in the lab in South Africa in 1955. Photograph courtesy of Dr. Henry Blackburn, University of Minnesota.

7.

THE FAT AND CHOLESTEROL HUMAN FEEDING STUDIES OF THE 1950S AND 1960S

What is amazing about Ancel Keys is that in addition to traveling the world performing the pre-studies and regular studies for the global epidemiological Seven Countries Study, he also maintained a full-fledged wet laboratory performing biological research at the University of Minnesota. This was before computers, email, faxes, and rapid travel by jet airplane–most of the trans-Atlantic travel for him and Margaret was carried out by ocean liner. After several population-based studies, Ancel Keys and his research group embarked in the 1950s on a series of highly controlled dietary feeding studies over a 10-year period in Minnesota that would precisely measure the effects of fat and other dietary constituents on blood cholesterol levels in men. If you read the papers closely, it is apparent how well these studies were designed with respect to the composition of the diets and the timings of the experiments. These studies, for the most part, were conducted in male schizophrenic patients that were housed in the Hastings State Hospital in Minnesota. These patients were treated with excellent medical care, and the food that was fed as part of the feeding studies was of the highest quality available and was skillfully prepared by knowledgeable cooks. An extensive experiment was reported in 1957 in the journal *Lancet*,[1] where the effects of dietary saturated, monounsaturated, and polyunsaturated fats, independently and together, were tested for their effects on blood cholesterol levels in men. The men were studied in groups of 12 to 27 and were fed the diets for two to nine weeks after a four-week standardization period. It was in this article that Dr. Keys published his "Keys equation," which showed that, when added to the diet, saturated fat raised and polyunsaturated fat lowered blood cholesterol in predictable ways, and that monounsaturated fats were neutral concerning the level of blood cholesterol.

A follow-up study, where Dr. Keys's laboratory measured 19 sets of comparisons, with 12 to 22 men in each set, was published in 1959 in the journal *Circulation*.[2] When the new studies were compared to the previous 41 sets of data, the "Keys equation" was still accurate in its ability to predict changes in blood cholesterol concentrations in groups of men in response to specific changes in fat type and content in the diets consumed.

In 1960 Dr. Keys and his laboratory group published a very interesting study in the *Journal of Nutrition* that investigated the role of other dietary constituents, besides the type and content of fat, on blood cholesterol concentrations.[3] This study was interesting because it tested the effects of a typical "American"

1. Keys A, Anderson JT, Grande F. (1957) Prediction of serum-cholesterol responses of man to changes in fats in the diet. *Lancet* 2: 959-966.
2. Keys A, Anderson JT, Grande F. (1959) Serum cholesterol in man: diet fat and intrinsic responsiveness. *Circulation* 19: 201-214. http://circ.ahajournals.org/content/19/2/201.long
3. Keys A, Anderson JT, Grande F. (1960) Diet-type (fats constant) and blood lipids in man. *J Nutrition* 70: 257-266. http://jn.nutrition.org/content/70/2/257.long

diet of the time versus a typical "Italian" diet. Both diets contained precisely controlled fat contents of either low- or moderate-fat levels. What is interesting is that Dr. Keys did not yet label the "Italian" diet he was testing the "Mediterranean" diet. That would come later, when he and Margaret published their third cook and health book, *How to Eat Well and Stay Well the Mediterranean Way.*[4] But this early study showed that Dr. Keys was coming to the conclusion that it was the Mediterranean diet as a whole, and not just the type and amount of fat consumed, that was protective against coronary heart disease.

The results from the *Journal of Nutrition* study were clear—in each case, whether the diets fed to the men contained low-fat or moderate-fat levels, blood cholesterol levels in the men were 15 to 20 mg/dL lower when the "Italian" type diet was consumed compared to when the typical "American" diet was consumed.

In the discussion Dr. Keys and colleagues wrote:

> The former (i.e, Italian or Mediterranean diet-inserted by the author) contained more fruits and vegetables of all kinds, especially dry legumes and green leafy vegetables, but was lower in sucrose, skim-milk solids and meat. The most likely cause of the difference between the effects of the diets would seem to be the difference in the nature of the carbohydrates or in some factors associated with carbohydrates such as cellulose, hemicelluloses or pectins. The diets producing lower serum cholesterol values were certainly higher in undigestible or difficultly digestible polysaccharides.[5]

The Protective Nature of Dietary Fiber, a Key Component in the Mediterranean Diet

Dr. Keys's comments on the likely role played by "cellulose,

4. Keys, A, Keys, M. (1975) *How to Eat Well and Stay Well the Mediterranean Way.* Garden City, New York: Doubleday & Company.
5. Ibid., page 264.

hemicelluloses or pectins" in the "Italian" type diet were prescient. In fact, the overall data that we have today on the protective properties of a high fiber intake against coronary heart disease are incredibly strong! The table below shows three examples from a larger group of studies that was used to set the fiber requirement for the 2005 U.S. Dietary Guidelines.

Table D5-1. Dietary Fiber Intake and Coronary Heart Disease (CHD): Prospective Cohort Studies

(The first 3 citations were used to establish AI for fiber in DRI Macronutrient report.)

Reference	Study Design	Quintile	Relative Risk for All or Fatal CHD	Dietary Fiber Intake (g/d)	Energy Intake (kcal/d)	Dietary Fiber Grams/1000 kcal
Pietinen et al., 1996	21,930 Finnish men, 50-69 y 6-y followup	1	1.00	16.1	2,722	5.9
		2	0.87	20.7	2,787	7.4
		3	0.78	24.3	2,781	8.7
		4	0.67	28.3	2,754	10.3
		5	0.68	34.8	2,705	12.9
			$P<0.001$			
Rimm et al., 1996	43,757 U.S. men, 40-75 y 6-y followup	1	1.00	12.4	2,000[a]	6.2
		2	0.97	16.6	2,000	8.3
		3	0.91	19.6	2,000	9.8
		4	0.87	23.0	2,000	11.5
		5	0.59	28.9	2,000	14.45
			$P<0.001$			
Wolk et al., 1999	68,782 U.S. women, 37-64y, 10-y followup	1	1.00	11.5	1,600[a]	7.2
		2	0.98	14.3	1,600	8.9
		3	0.92	16.4	1,600	10.25
		4	0.87	18.8	1,600	11.75
		5	0.77	22.9	1,600	14.31
			$P=0.07$			

http://www.health.gov/dietaryguidelines/dga2005/report/HTML/table_d5_1.htm

The full references for each study can be found in the Dietary Guidelines report found in the link. The term "AI" refers to Adequate Intake, which is the Dietary Reference Intake (DRI) parameter used for dietary fiber. The red arrows (placed by the author) show the protective effect at the highest fiber intake in each group. The value for significance in each study is for the trend; therefore the lesser amounts of fiber are protective but the higher amounts are more protective.

The data in this table[6] are interesting and extremely relevant because there was a dose effect of fiber intake in each study, and

6. http://www.health.gov/dietaryguidelines/dga2005/report/HTML/table_d5_1.htm

the protective effects on CHD were especially strong at the higher doses of fiber in each study. Also extremely important, the dose effect of fiber was observed in both men and women. There is much debate among scientists concerning which type of fiber is more beneficial in the protection against coronary heart disease.[7] Many individual studies have noted protection of fiber against coronary heart disease when both men and women were analyzed[8] or when men alone were studied.[9] A comparative analysis of studies in the literature was recently published where an expanded definition of fiber was used, such that intakes of bran, germ, generic fiber and whole grain foods were allowed, and a total of 29 studies were included in the comparisons. The results were that, in a majority of the studies, consistent beneficial, protective effects against coronary heart disease, or markers associated with coronary heart disease, were observed when the diet contained higher levels of fiber.[10]

One possible way that dietary fiber could be influencing coronary heart disease is by causing small changes in the excretion of cholesterol and its metabolites in the stool. Effects of fiber on excretion of cholesterol or its metabolites could make a great difference in overall cholesterol metabolism in the body

7. Mobley AR, Jones JM, Rodriguez J, Slavin J, Zelman KM. (2014) Identifying practical solutions to meet America's fiber needs: proceedings from the Food & Fiber Summit. *Nutrients* 6(7): 2540-2551. http://www.mdpi.com/2072-6643/6/7/2540
8. Steffen LM, Jacobs DR Jr, Stevens J, Shahar E, Carithers T, Folsom AR. (2003) Associations of whole-grain, refined-grain, and fruit and vegetable consumption with risks of all-cause mortality and incident coronary artery disease and ischemic stroke: the Atherosclerosis Risk in Communities (ARIC) Study. *Am J Clin Nutr* 78(3): 383-390. http://ajcn.nutrition.org/content/78/3/383.long
9. Jensen MK, Koh-Banerjee P, Hu FB, Franz M, Sampson L, Grønbaek M, Rimm EB. (2004) Intakes of whole grains, bran, and germ and the risk of coronary heart disease in men. *Am J Clin Nutr* 80(6): 1492-1499. http://ajcn.nutrition.org/content/80/6/1492.long
10. De Moura FF, Lewis KD, Falk MC. (2009) Applying the FDA definition of whole grains to the evidence for cardiovascular disease health claims. *J Nutr* 139(11):2220S-2226S. http://jn.nutrition.org/content/139/11/2220S.long

over the long term. However, it is not certain that this is the mechanism of the beneficial effects of fiber because studies performed in humans measuring the effects of dietary fiber on cholesterol excretion have been relatively short term in duration. Also, because the analytical methods at the time were not powerful enough to measure altered metabolites, many of the earlier balance studies may have missed other chemical species of cholesterol and bile acids that were formed during intestinal metabolism and then excreted in the stool. It is still amazing to me that the health effects of dietary fiber are not stressed in the media or promoted by doctors or medical associations.

In 1965 Dr. Keys published a series of four articles in the journal *Metabolism* that reviewed all of the human feeding studies that addressed the effects of diet on blood cholesterol concentration.[11] [12] [13] [14] In these papers Dr. Keys summed up the feeding studies he had performed in Minnesota over the preceding 10-year period, and he compared them to the studies that had been conducted by other investigators. In extensive comments and discussion, Dr. Keys described the details of the experiments and provided data that supported the accuracy of the Keys equation.

About 10 years after the *Metabolism* articles had appeared, and after he had retired, Dr. Keys published an additional study that addressed the question of whether the amount of cholesterol itself in the diet was important in controlling the concentration

11. Keys A, Anderson JT, Grande F. (1965) Serum cholesterol responses to changes in the diet. I. Iodine value of dietary fat versus 2S-P. *Metabolism* 14: 747-758. http://www.ncbi.nlm.nih.gov/pubmed/?term=PMID%3A+++++25286459
12. Keys A, Anderson JT, Grande F. (1965) Serum cholesterol responses to changes in the diet. II. The effect of cholesterol in the diet. *Metabolism* 14: 759-765. http://www.ncbi.nlm.nih.gov/pubmed/25286460
13. Keys A, Anderson JT, Grande F. (1965) Serum cholesterol responses to changes in the diet. III. Differences among individuals. *Metabolism* 14: 766-775. http://www.ncbi.nlm.nih.gov/pubmed/25286465
14. Keys A, Anderson JT, Grande F. (1965) Serum cholesterol responses to changes in the diet. IV. Particular saturated fatty acids in the diet. *Metabolism* 14: 776-787. http://www.ncbi.nlm.nih.gov/pubmed/25286466

of cholesterol in blood.[15] What was observed in this last feeding study was that increasing the amount of cholesterol in the diet, from practically zero to the amount usually found in the American diet (approximately 300 to 400 mg of cholesterol per day), increased blood cholesterol only by about 7 to 8 mg of cholesterol/dL. These effects of dietary cholesterol on blood cholesterol concentration were small in comparison to the effects previously observed for saturated fat. However, an increase in 7 to 8 mg of cholesterol/dL is still significant when considering very large populations. The 1976 study published by Dr. Keys supported earlier experiments that had been performed in the Keys's lab[16] but had been criticized by several scientists as being inadequate because their own results had showed a greater response to dietary cholesterol. Dr. Keys concisely wrote in one earlier article, "We, therefore, conclude that the effects on serum cholesterol of changing the amount or nature of the dietary fat were independent of the amount of cholesterol in the diet."[17] In one of the papers in the *Metabolism* series, Dr. Keys had also commented, "For the purpose of controlling the serum level, dietary cholesterol should not be completely ignored but attention to this factor alone accomplished little."[18] The later 1976 article by Anderson JT, Grande F, and Keys A. (1976), definitely showed that the previous cholesterol feeding studies had been correct and accurate.

We have to remember that at this time (1976), Dr. Keys did

15. Anderson JT, Grande F, Keys A. (1976) Independence of the effects of cholesterol and degree of saturation of the fat in the diet on serum cholesterol in man. *Am J Clin Nutrition* 29: 1184-1189. http://ajcn.nutrition.org/content/29/11/1184.long
16. Grande F, Anderson JT, Chlouverakis C, Proja M, Keys A. (1965) Effect of Dietary Cholesterol on Man's Serum Lipids. *J Nutrition* 87: 52-62. http://www.ncbi.nlm.nih.gov/pubmed/?term=5834575
17. Ibid., page 61.
18. Keys A, Anderson JT, Grande F. (1965) Serum cholesterol responses to changes in the diet. II. The effect of cholesterol in the diet. *Metabolism* 14: 759-765, page 759.

not have access to the very large data sets that measured the effects of small changes in blood cholesterol concentration, in combination with other individual risk factors, on the overall risk for coronary heart disease. Nonetheless, the extremely well executed experiments performed in Dr. Keys's laboratory on the effects of diet (fat type, inclusion of fiber, and dietary cholesterol content) on blood cholesterol would stand the test of time and greatly improve the health of Americans in the following decades.

In summary, through carefully executed feeding studies performed in his laboratory at the University of Minnesota, and through far reaching, global epidemiological studies, Dr. Ancel Keys and his research group not only determined the precise effects of dietary fat and cholesterol on blood cholesterol concentrations, he also determined that the "Italian" diet, later referred to as the Mediterranean diet, contained multiple components that protected against coronary heart disease. Both his laboratory studies, and his long trek around the globe in search of ecological and dietary factors that conveyed beneficial effects on health, led Ancel and Margaret Keys in 1975 to publish their health promoting masterpiece, *How to Eat Well and Stay Well the Mediterranean Way.*

8.

AFTER SEVEN COUNTRIES-RETIREMENT, LIFE IN ITALY, AND SCIENTIFIC LEGACY

After leading the Seven Countries Study, Ancel Keys had accumulated four very large and significant accomplishments that highlight a remarkable scientific career. These accomplishments were:

1. Formulated ready-to-eat meals (called K rations) for the American armed forces during World War II;
2. Studied starvation for the purpose of learning the best procedures for treating starved individuals;
3. Conceived and implemented the Seven Countries Study that pointed to diet as being an important factor in the development of coronary heart disease; and

4. Performed extensive human feeding studies that led to the formulation of the "Keys Equation."

Dr. Keys's and Margaret's travels during the Seven Countries Study convinced him that the Mediterranean diet was an important factor in maintaining health. With this knowledge, Dr. Keys and Margaret, a biochemist, wrote three very popular cookbooks that would help people eat healthy. These were *Eat Well and Stay Well* (1959),[1] and an updated version, *How to Eat Well and Stay Well the Mediterranean Way* (1975).[2] Both books were featured on the *New York Times* best seller list. They wrote a third book, *The Benevolent Bean*, published in 1967, and it was also successful.[3] A collage of the covers of the three books is shown below:

1. Keys A, Keys M. (1959) *Eat Well and Stay Well.* Garden City, New York: Doubleday & Company.
2. Keys A, Keys M. (1975) How to Eat Well and Stay Well the Mediterranean Way. Garden City, New York: Doubleday & Company
3. Keys A, Keys M. (1967) The Benevolent Bean. Garden City, New York: Doubleday & Company. Edition I read: Noonday Edition, 1972, New York: Noonday Press, a division of Farrar, Straus and Giroux.

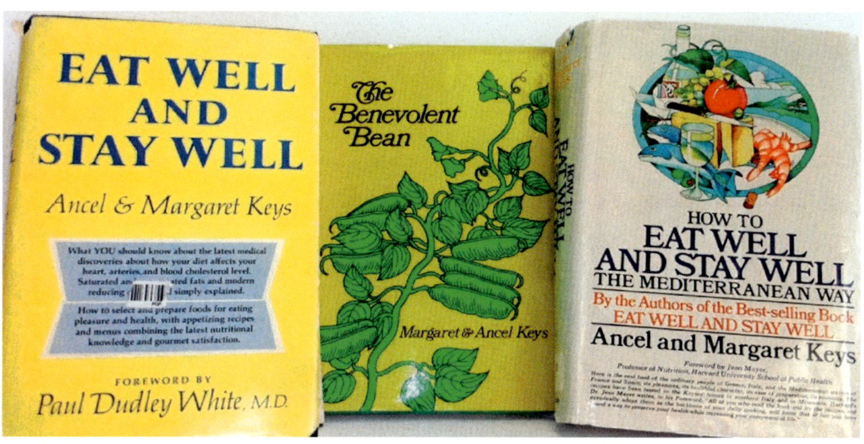

The covers of the three cookbooks written by Ancel and Margaret Keys. Photograph of the collage by JL Dixon. The cover images were used by permission of Penguin Random House LLC (which Doubleday & Company, Inc. is now part of) and Farrar, Straus and Giroux, LLC (which published The Benevolent Bean in 1972). The rights are fully explained in the Updates section.

Rick Ashford of the *Minnesota Daily* newspaper wrote on March 6, 1959, "Their new book, *Eat Well and Stay Well*, to be published March 19th, is the best bargain on the market (3.95) for the seeker after healthful nutrients."[4] The entire book was serialized in the *Minnesota Star* newspaper during the spring of 1959.[5] The April 17, 1959, post from *Eat Well and Stay Well* was entitled, *Don't Depend on Meat Alone,* by Dr. and Mrs. Ancel Keys. A quote from Dr. Keys in the section introduction was: "Sausage is pure 'Baloney' as far as high fat content is concerned."

In *Eat Well and Stay Well,*[6] the Keys summarized their advice with these sensible recommendations:

1. Do not get fat, if you are fat, reduce.

4. Ashford R, (1959) *Minnesota Daily* newspaper, March 6, 1959.
5. Keys A, Keys M. (1959) Don't Depend on Meat Alone. *Minnesota Star,* April 17, 1959.
6. Keys A, Keys M. (1959) *Eat Well and Stay Well,* page 40.

2. Restrict saturated fats, the fats in beef, pork, lamb, sausages, margarine, solid shortenings, fats in dairy products.
3. Prefer vegetable oils to solid fats, but keep total fats under 30% of your diet calories.
4. Favor fresh vegetables, fruits, and non-fat milk products.
5. Avoid heavy use of salt and refined sugar.
6. Good diets do not depend upon drugs and fancy preparations.
7. Get plenty of exercise and outdoor recreation.
8. Be sensible about cigarettes, alcohol, excitement, business strain.
9. See your doctor regularly and do not worry.

These recommendations, made in 1959, foreshadowed those of the dietary guidelines by about 20 years.

Interestingly, there was some push back from the agriculture sector. The following is a review of *Eat Well and Stay Well* by Ancel and Margaret Keys that I found in the official Ancel Keys archives at the University of Minnesota. This review appeared in the May 1959 issue of *Food and Nutrition News*,[7] a serial publication of the National Live Stock and Meat Board.

> EAT WELL AND STAY WELL by Ancel and Margaret Keys. Doubleday and Co., Garden City, N.Y., 1959. Pp. 359 $3.95.
>
> (Par. 1.) Dr. Keys, a renowned physiologist, and his wife, a biochemist, have collaborated on this combination nutrition text and cookbook which is designed for physicians and laymen.
>
> (Par. 2.) The book's title may be somewhat misleading. To the authors "staying well" apparently means not dying of heart disease or atherosclerosis. Many persons do not have either conditions, but nevertheless are not well because they do not eat well.

7. "Review of Eat Well and Stay Well," in *Food and Nutrition News* 30(8): 3-4, May 1959, published by the National Live Stock and Meat Board. A version of this review typed on plain white paper was found among Dr. Keys's papers in: University of Minnesota Archives-Visited August 2014. Ancel B. Keys papers, Creator: Keys, Ancel Benjamin, 1904-2004; Repository: University of Minnesota Libraries, Elmer L. Andersen Library, uar@umn.edu; Collection Number: uarc 738 https://www.lib.umn.edu/special/gettingarchives

(Par. 3.) It is doubtful that the Keys will find much support among nutritionists, dietitians, physicians, and other professionals persons regarding dietary recommendations. Actually, it is difficult to determine what the book does recommend. It seems to recommend a nutritionally adequate diet, but then proceeds to indict each of the food groups that make up such a diet. In the end you feel that the only food items the authors really approve of are wine, home-made Italian bread, skim milk, cottage cheese and vegetable oils.

(Par. 4.) Tables of food composition are featured on the jacket of the book and the foreward. In these tables the calorie, fat and protein values for meat are given on the raw, edible portion only. Recent research findings would present a much more accurate picture–for physicians as well as laymen–of the nutrient content of meat as it is produced and eaten today.

(Par. 5.) Certain inaccuracies in the text have been noticed. Riboflavin is said to be "abundant" in whole grains, meats, etc. An average serving of cereal (1/2 cup) would provide 2.2 per cent of the recommended daily intake for a man. This could hardly be considered abundant. (One serving of beef provides 21.7 per cent.) Haddock and sardines are incorrectly compared with hamburger as sources of protein. The statement is made that in hamburger steak 75 per cent of the calories are from fat. The fat content (in calories) ranges from 21.1 to 58.1 per cent.

(Par. 6.) The recipe and menu sections account for more than half of this book and, therefore, will be of considerable interest to those who purchase it. We wonder why, in a book supposedly aimed at nutritional well being, nine pages are devoted to wine and alcoholic beverages, and 16 pages to desserts, five to eggs, and only ten to meats (including rabbit).

(Par. 7.) Certain meat cookery methods included in the book are extreme departures from the recommendations of recognized authorities in the field of home economics.

This was an interesting review of *Eat Well and Stay Well*! The comment comparing protein in haddock and sardines to protein in hamburger (Par. 5) is especially questionable. Dr. Keys knew, without a doubt, that fish was a healthier source of protein and nutrients than hamburger!

Kay Savage, the food editor of the *Detroit Free Press*, wrote the following in her September 11, 1967, review [8] of the *Benevolent Bean*: "One unique feature of their book, published by Doubleday & Co. at $3.95, is the calorie, protein and fat count at the end of each recipe." And, "Tracing the history and the food value of beans, the Keys' bring to light many interesting facts. Yet, the nutritional information is not on the clinical level, and the many recipes offered in the book are bound to make you want to head for the kitchen and start cooking."

Interestingly, the success of the cookbooks allowed Dr. Keys and his wife to move to the town of Pioppi, south of Naples, Italy, to live during their retirement and eat a Mediterranean diet up close and personal all year long. The picture below is a view of the village of Pioppi as it now appears. The Keyses' house was north of the town, right up from the shore, on the hill shown in the left background. When the Keyses lived in Pioppi, it was much smaller and less crowded. Their life in Italy will be described below and in the last few chapters.

8. Savage K, (1967) *Detroit Free Press*, September 11, 1967.

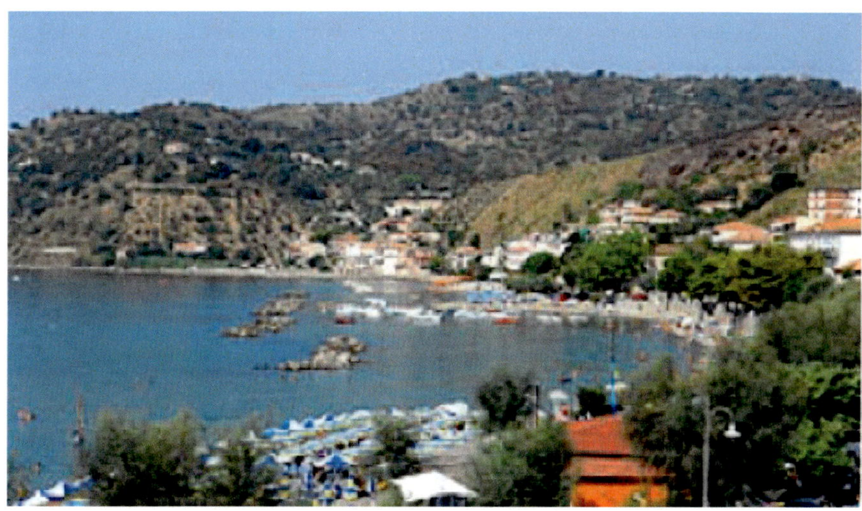

View of the Italian coastline near village of Pioppi, Italy, from a travel website (http://www.emmeti.it/Welcome/Campania/Salernitano/Pioppi/index.uk.html) This is a favorite view of Pioppi seen in many travel brochures and websites.

In my mind, the cookbooks that Ancel and Margaret Keys wrote were another major accomplishment in their careers, because through these books and newspaper articles, millions of people improved their health by eating a Mediterranean diet.

After his retirement from the University of Minnesota (at the time, faculty were forced to retire at age 67), Dr. Keys continued as an emeritus professor, but he and Margaret spent more and more time in southern Italy.

Ancel Keys tracked the data from the participants in the Seven Countries Study for several follow-ups, but after retiring, he settled down to direct the writing of the famous book, *Seven Countries*, which was published in 1980 by Harvard University Press. Preliminary reports on the baseline data and the five-year experiences of the Seven Countries Study had been published in several monographs and in journals.[9] [10]

In an article in the *St. Paul Pioneer Press* on May 21, 1973,[11] the interviewer caught Dr. and Mrs. Keys getting ready to leave for Europe. Some of the interesting quotes from this article were: "He took a lot of heat from the dairy industry over the years for his recommendations that margarine should be used instead of butter; skim milk instead of whole...My objection to the customary diet is that it's high in saturated fats, meats, and sugar. Those should be reduced in most people's diet."

In this interview Dr. Keys also commented on the Atkins diet: "The only new kicker is Atkins's suggestion that escaping ketones drastically eliminate body fat. Studies have shown that the most ketones that the body can eliminate a day is 100 mg., a quite small amount." When I read this I immediately thought of Dr. Keys's thorough studies into starvation during World War II, when he observed that individuals suffering from severe ketosis "were in real bad shape." Due to his groundbreaking studies into starvation, I imagine it is an understatement to say that Ancel Keys would have known a fair amount about the effects of ketosis on the human body!

A later interview with Dr. Keys by William Hoffman was published in the March 1979 issue of "Update," a quarterly publication from the Department of University Relations at the University of Minnesota.[12] This interview contained several historically important statements, and must have been conducted by phone, as it found Dr. Keys finishing the book on the Seven

9. Keys A, Aravanis C, Blackburn H, Van Buchem FSP, Buzina R, Djordjević BS, Dontas AS, Fidanza F, Karvonen MJ, Kimura N, Lekos D, Monti M, Puddu V, Taylor HL. (1967) Epidemiological studies related to coronary heart disease. Characteristics of men aged 40-59 in Seven Countries. *Acta Med Scand* 460(Suppl.180):392 pp.
10. Keys A (Ed). (1970) Coronary heart disease in seven countries. *Circulation* 41(Suppl.1):211 pp.
11. *St. Paul Pioneer Press,* May 21, 1973. Found as a clipping in the Ancel Keys Archives in the University of Minnesota Archives at the Elmer L. Andersen Library.
12. Hoffman, W. (1979) "Meet Monsieur Cholesterol" (Profile of world renowned cardiovascular epidemiologist Ancel Keys). *Update* (University of Minnesota). http://mbbnet.umn.edu/hoff/hoff_ak.html

Countries Study that would be published soon. Mr. Hoffman wrote, "He walks and swims a lot in Italy – but has no intention of joining up with the joggers." He quoted Dr. Keys, "Margaret and I get lots of pleasure from working in our yard. We just started the olive harvest. We have 80 olive trees and 75 citrus trees. We have oranges, tangerines, apricots, pears — lots of pears — plums, and four apple trees that produced only one apple so far. Also we have kumquats and chinotto. You probably don't know about chinotto. It's a citrus fruit, redder than most tangerines, and it grows on a beautiful tree. Produces lots of wonderful fruit for marmalade."

There were some questions about the K rations, and Mr. Hoffman quoted Dr. Keys as saying, "Six months later, I went down to Fort Benning, Georgia, to run more elaborate trials. Then General McNair, the chief of infantry at the time, said that *this* was going to be the combat ration because it was easy to hand out. The logistics were simple, that's all. But I was surprised when I saw the packages start to roll in with 'K' on them. Then I got a letter from Colonel Logan of the Quartermaster Corps in Washington saying he hoped I wouldn't mind."

There were some questions in the interview on the Keyses' life in Italy. Dr. Keys said, "When we started off on this last trip we had to get a young fellow to drive us to Rome because the railroad was on strike." The Keyses' home was about a four-hour drive south of Naples and near a fishing village. "We come back to Minnesota for July and August, primarily because our little village swells from 500 people to 4,500 during the tourist season...Not long ago, when we bought our house, the roads were poor and there were no hotels in the south of Italy."

What I found very interesting about this interview–published in March 1979–was that there were no comments concerning the Dietary Guidelines that were in the news in the United States in 1979 and 1980. In fact, one of the reasons I traveled to Minnesota to look through the Ancel Keys archives was to search for information concerning Dr. Keys's role in the development of the Dietary Guidelines. In my nine hours of going through his files, both in the University of Minnesota Archives at the Elmer L. Andersen Library and at the Division of Epidemiology, I did not find one letter, note, or even word referring to the Dietary Guidelines. There is no evidence that Dr. Keys participated in any of the government deliberations leading to the U.S. Dietary Guidelines. Dr. Keys, having retired and living in Italy most of this time, was far removed from the whole process, and he was probably working on the final version of the book that was scheduled to be published in 1980.

To illustrate the difficulties that Dr. and Margaret Keys encountered in working overseas, I have paraphrased a much longer, extremely funny story that I found in the Division of Epidemiology archives: "A computer arrives in Italy," by Margaret Keys.[13]

In August 1984 Dr. Keys asked the Italian authorities if he needed documents to send his computer from Minnesota to Italy to continue writing at his home, Minnelea. He learned that he would need an import license. Furthermore, a permit was required to use the computer in Italy. Incredibly, the permit was good for only one year and it was not renewable.

After negotiations between the University of Minnesota and Italy, the computer was sent with an import tax to be paid upon its arrival at the airport. The computer was shipped on September 13 and arrived at the airport on November 26 in 9 boxes, and the import tax was $1,350! The next day Dr. Keys and Martii Karvonen drove to the airport to pick up the computer.

But they couldn't pick it up because they were told a document, "Benestare Bancaria," which could only be obtained from a bank in Salerno, was required. Upon arriving at the bank, they learned they needed another document, "Codice Fiscale," to obtain the

13. Archives of Dr. Ancel Keys and Margaret Keys, and the Seven Countries Study. University of Minnesota Division of Epidemiology and Community Health. Courtesy of Dr. H Blackburn. http://www.epi.umn.edu/cvdepi/

"Benestare Bancaria." They needed to drive to Vallo della Lucania to obtain the "Codice Fiscale," and then return for the "Benestare Bancaria." After they obtained both documents, they proceeded to the airport where they were told the customs office was too busy to help them. They returned the next day and picked up the boxes, but learned later the computer console was absent. On December 22 the final box was brought to Minnelea by Jerry and Rose Stamler, who had picked it up from Dr. Mario Mancini in Naples.

By January 9, 1985, a technician from DEC had installed the computer and it was working. This was the escapade written about with such comic relief by Margaret Keys, greatly abbreviated here, that was required to bring a computer to Italy for Dr. Keys to work on! This unpublished article offers readers insights into Margaret Keys's sense of humor!

In 1986, Dr. Keys was first author on an article that related to the 15-year follow-up of the Seven Countries Study.[14] Other articles that were published by Dr. Keys, or more recently by his colleagues, can be found on the Seven Countries website: http://sevencountriesstudy.com/study-findings/publications

Scientific Legacy of Ancel Keys

During the first half of the 20th century, deaths from cardiovascular diseases were increasing in the United States. This is shown in the next figure, which is from an article that was written by a special panel of experts reporting from the *National Conference on Cardiovascular Disease Prevention,* held September 1999, and published in the journal *Circulation.*[15] Deaths from a

14. Keys A, Menotti A, Karvonen MJ, Aravanis C, Blackburn H, Buzina R, Djordjevic BS, Dontas AS, Fidanza F, Keys MH, et al. (1986) The diet and 15-year death rate in the seven countries study. *Am J Epidemiol.* 124(6): 903-15.
15. Cooper R, Cutler J, Desvigne-Nickens P, Fortmann SP, Friedman L, Havlik R, Hogelin G, Marler J, McGovern P, Morosco G, Mosca L, Pearson T, Stamler J,

variety of vascular diseases (except stroke) increased during the first half of the century, with peaks occurring around the 40s to the early 60s. Dr. Ancel Keys decided to study this phenomenon and take action. The Seven Countries Study led to valuable insights into the connections between diet and lifestyle and coronary heart disease. With the new knowledge concerning the role of dietary saturated fat in enhancing blood cholesterol levels, and other factors such as dietary fiber that protected against coronary heart disease, the rates of coronary heart disease and other cardiovascular conditions were slowed and then started to decline (see figure).

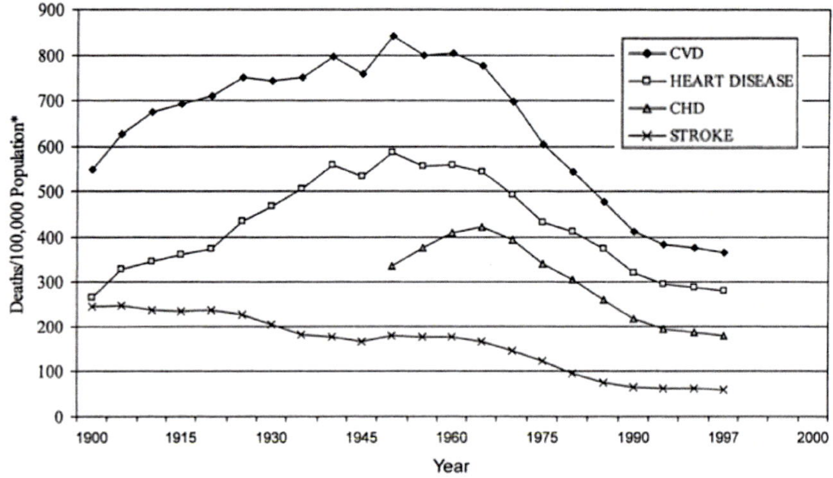

Cooper R. et al. (2000) Trends and disparities in coronary heart disease... *Circulation* 102(25): 3137-3147. http://circ.ahajournals.org/content/102/25/3137.long

Stryer D, Thom T. (2000) Trends and disparities in coronary heart disease, stroke, and other cardiovascular diseases in the United States: findings of the national conference on cardiovascular disease prevention. *Circulation* 102(25): 3137-3147. http://circ.ahajournals.org/content/102/25/3137.long

Starting about 1965, the rates began to drop and continued to decrease throughout the remaining years of the century. These decreases were the result of the war against cardiovascular disease that was initiated by Dr. Ancel Keys of the University of Minnesota, the staff and doctors of the National Heart, Lung, and Blood Institute of NIH, and a host of other researchers in the cardiovascular disease field.

The final question concerning the blood cholesterol/coronary heart disease connection was whether cholesterol lowering, especially LDL cholesterol lowering, would be accompanied by a decrease in coronary heart disease, and whether this observation could be confirmed using the gold standard study: a randomized, double-blind intervention trial. In the early 1970s, Dr. Theodoroe Cooper, Director of the National Heart, Lung, and Blood Institute, was determined to answer this question. First, a series of "Lipid Research Clinics" were established to provide standardized lipid measurements and expertise to large intervention trials. In 1971 an expert panel was asked to design a study that would be powerful enough to provide a definitive answer, one way or the other, whether LDL cholesterol lowering decreased coronary heart disease. Dr. Daniel Steinberg was the co-chair of this panel, and he described in great detail in his book, *The Cholesterol Wars,*[16] the deliberations that led to the design of this 13-year, $150 million study. After two years of planning the design of the study was settled on. In order to recruit the 3,800 men with blood cholesterol concentrations over 265, almost 500,000 men were screened. A major role in the recruitment process was played by Dr. Gustave Schonfeld, who was director of the Lipid Research Clinic at Washington University in St. Louis.[17] The full cohort was recruited in 1976 and the clinical portion of the study continued until each participant had been followed for at least 5 years. The

16. Steinberg D. (2007) *The Cholesterol Wars, The Skeptics vs. the Preponderance of Evidence.* Amsterdam: Academic Press (Elsevier), page 145.
17. Ibid., page 148.

question was answered in January 1984 when the results of the National Heart, Lung, and Blood Institute's Lipid Research Clinics Coronary Primary Prevention Trial were published.[18] In this study, 3,806 asymptomatic middle-aged men with primary hypercholesterolemia were either treated with a bile acid sequestrant (cholestyramine resin) or received a placebo (the control group) for an average of 7.4 years. Both groups were instructed to consume a moderate cholesterol-lowering diet.

When the study was finally published the results were extremely exciting. The cholestyramine group experienced a 24% reduction in definite coronary heart disease death and a 19% reduction in nonfatal myocardial infarction. The many years that Dr. Keys and his team had labored performing ecological epidemiological and cholesterol-feeding studies to bring clarity to the diet/blood cholesterol/coronary heart disease connection would be supported with the gold standard scientific epidemiological study: the randomized, double-blind intervention trial. No longer would there be doubt concerning whether a high blood LDL cholesterol concentration increased the risk for coronary heart disease. The National Heart, Lung, and Blood Institute's Lipid Research Clinics Coronary Primary Prevention Trial results would confirm with certainty what many scientists had suspected for many years. Also, the results of this carefully designed and rigorously carried out study would finally ameliorate those who were skeptical of the "cholesterol hypothesis"–at least the skeptics who were somewhat logical!

18. Many Authors (1984) The Lipid Research Clinics Coronary Primary Prevention Trial Results I. Reduction in Incidence of Coronary Heart Disease. *Journal of the American Medical Association* 251(3): 351-364.

9.

A SUCCESSFUL COLLABORATION CONTINUES THE SEVEN COUNTRIES STUDY

When Dr. Keys underwent forced retirement at the University of Minnesota in 1972 at the age of 67, Dr. Henry Blackburn, who had started as an intern in 1953 and was appointed to a permanent position at the University of Minnesota in 1956, was chosen to head the Laboratory of Physiological Hygiene. In 1983, he facilitated its merger with epidemiology to create the Division of Epidemiology and Community Health in the School of Public Health.

A Visit to the University of Minnesota to View the Ancel Keys and Seven Countries Study Archives

I traveled to the University of Minnesota to visit the Ancel Keys archives. First, I visited the Ancel Keys archives at the Elmer L. Andersen Library. Later in the day, I met Dr. Blackburn in his office at the Division of Epidemiology and Community Health in the School of Public Health on the campus of the university. I was amazed at the man I encountered, because I hope very much to have the level of energy and clarity when I am 89 years old that Dr. Blackburn exhibited during my visit! We had a wonderful two-hour conversation that spanned his 60 years of experiences as a participant and co-leader of the Seven Countries Study. I had brought a series of questions with me and he answered every one of them completely and with enthusiasm. I then made plans to visit the next day to go through the files of Dr. Ancel Keys and the Seven Countries Study.

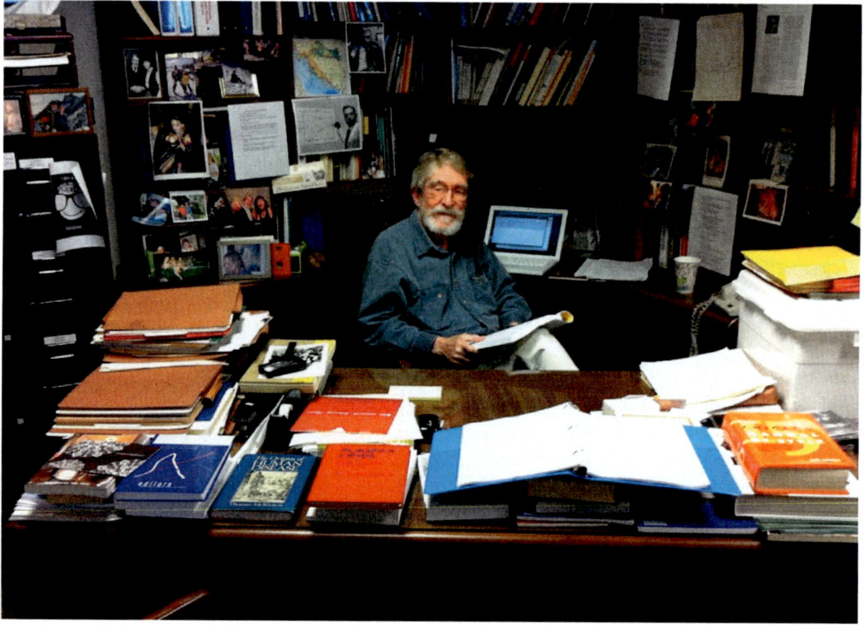

Dr. Henry Blackburn, August 2014, at his desk at the University of Minnesota Division of Epidemiology and Community Health. Photograph by JL Dixon.

The next morning I arrived at the Division of Epidemiology and started my journey through the life of Ancel Keys and the 60 years of the Seven Countries Study. The files at the division headquarters were much more extensive than those in the Andersen Library, and the four hours I had allotted for this part of the journey were ridiculously too short, but I had come with specific questions I wished to have answered. I could have spent a month there! However, the files of Dr. Keys are meticulously organized, and there is an extensive Excel spreadsheet that shows how the files are organized in each cabinet, so that it was quite easy to go directly to the episode or study that I was looking for.

Below are pictures of the area where the files of the Seven Countries Study are kept at the Division of Epidemiology and Community Medicine. On the cabinets near the windows are books that were written by scientists who participated in the study. In the second picture, the colorful picture of Ancel Keys is the cover of *Time* magazine from 1961. On the cabinets on the right side are a series of books with blue covers. These are all the scientific papers that were published from the Laboratory of Physiological Hygiene (and later the Division of Epidemiology) from the years 1937 to about 1989. A close-up of these bound articles is in the third picture.

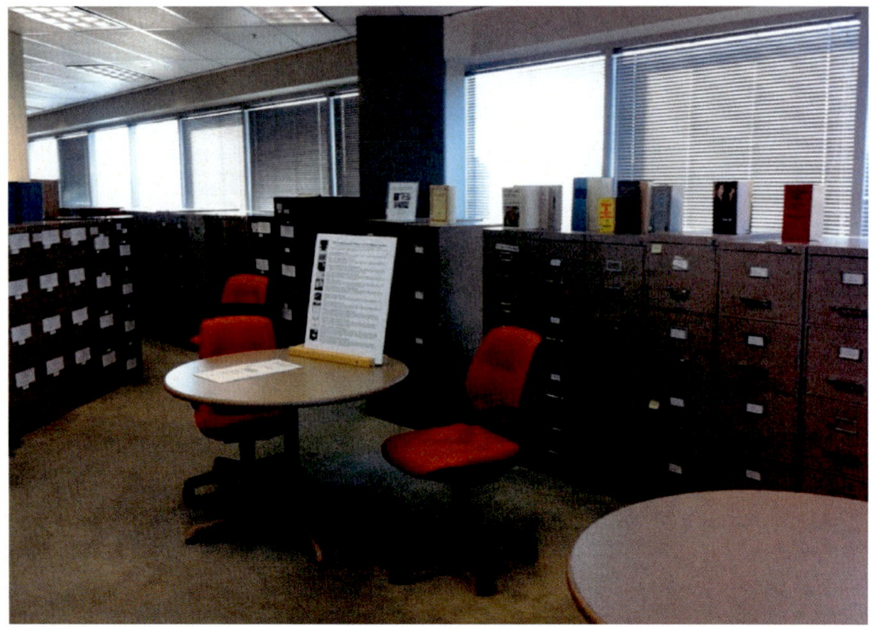

Files and books from the Seven Countries Study, Division of Epidemiology and Community Health, University of Minnesota. Photograph by JL Dixon, August 2014.

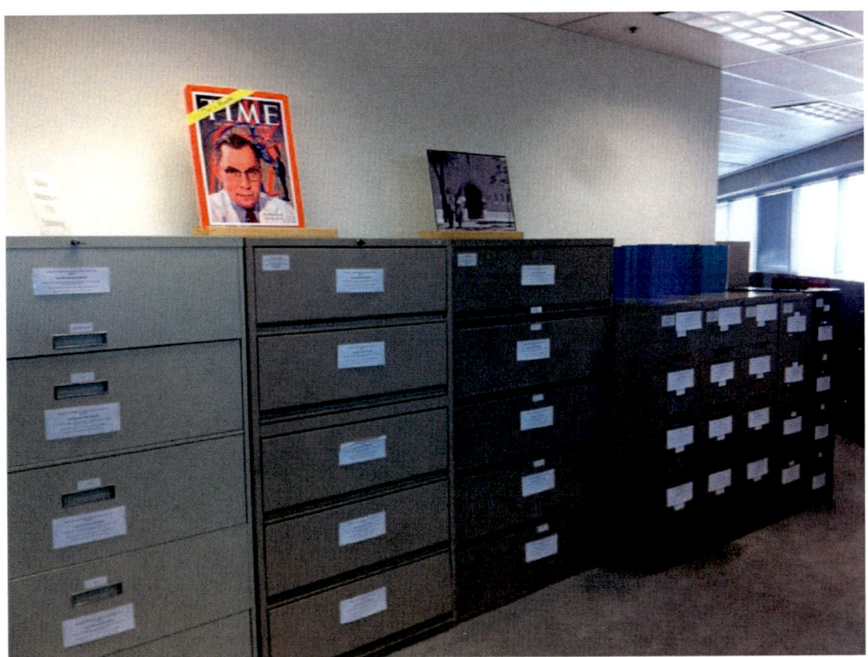

On top of cabinets: Time cover of Dr. Ancel Keys and bound papers from the Laboratory of Physiological Hygiene. Photograph by JL Dixon, August 2014.

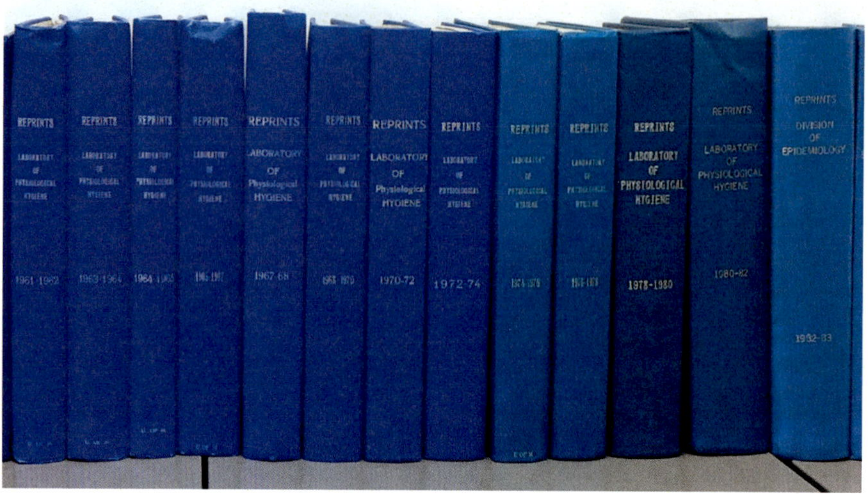

Close-up of a portion of the bound reprints from the Laboratory of Physiological Hygiene. Now kept at the Division of Epidemiology and Community Medicine, School of Public Health, University of Minnesota. Photograph by JL Dixon, August 2014.

The science that was performed in the Seven Countries Study is published in over 500 articles in scientific journals and in a series of monographs. I had already read many of these and, therefore, I had a strong foundation (I hoped) in the science. What I was looking for were answers to specific questions that I had brought with me to Minnesota.

One has to remember that Dr. Keys's research and the Seven Countries Study set into motion a complex series of studies that led to many other scientific investigations. Beyond the bound scientific papers that emanated from the University of Minnesota's Laboratory of Physiological Hygiene are hundreds of scientific articles that were published by scientists from the target countries who participated as colleagues in the Seven Countries Study.

When a media nutrition expert takes a paragraph from one particular paper and uses that paragraph to cast suspicion on 60 years of research, it is like looking at one poorly cut block of the Great Pyramid of Khufu at Giza and stating that the structure was poorly designed and improperly built. It defies logic and fairness when someone who has no comprehension of the scientific method attacks years of hard work and dedication.

One of the most surprising experiences of my life occurred when I asked Dr. Blackburn for copies of three documents that I found especially interesting, and he quickly and graciously went off to personally copy the documents for me.

Dr. Blackburn started his professional career at the Laboratory of Physiological Hygiene by collaborating in a study in the United States being led by Dr. Henry Longstreet Taylor, one of the professors at the lab. This story is described by Dr. Blackburn in chapter four of the 1994 monograph.[1]

Dr. Taylor's idea was to "compare coronary heart disease (CHD) rates among men with different rail occupations to get at the causal role of habitual physical activity."[2] Dr. Taylor proposed to study active switchmen compared to relatively inactive clerks. The National Institutes of Health (NIH) review committee liked his idea and the NIH funded the U.S. Railroad (USRR) Study. This study started before the official Seven Countries Study, but the methods it developed, and in fact, the later portions of the USRR study itself, became part of the Seven Countries Study.

Dr. Blackburn's role was to develop the diagnostic methods for the railroad study and he also worked with Dr. Taylor in the design of the Pullman railroad car, which would be converted into a rolling clinic that included rooms for physical exams, performing resting and exercise electrocardiography, an X-ray

1. Blackburn, H. Chapter 4. "Studies in the U.S. Railroad." pages 45-55. In: Kromhout D, Menotti A, Blackburn H (Eds). *(1994) The Seven Countries Study: A scientific adventure in cardiovascular disease epidemiology.* Brouwer Offset b.v., Utrecht, ISBN 90-6960-048-x, 219 pp. This and other monographs and references can be found on the Seven Countries Study website: http://sevencountriesstudy.com/study-findings/publications
2. Ibid., page 45.

booth, and a full wet laboratory for processing blood samples. The Pullman traveling clinic was attached to trains that traveled throughout the entire railway system designated for the study, and it soon visited sites and towns throughout the Midwest and West, including St. Louis, Seattle, Portland, San Francisco, and then back to Minneapolis.

One of the important lessons from the USRR study was the concept that many more subjects were needed to be recruited into individual cohorts in order to have enough cases of disease develop in a reasonable follow-up period. The main scientific take home message of the USRR study was that lack of physical activity was a weaker risk factor for coronary heart disease than blood cholesterol or systolic blood pressure.[3 4]

The procedures, disease classification system, and forms developed in the USRR study were later used in the Seven Countries Study when it officially began in Dalmatia in the fall of 1958.

After Dr. Keys retired in 1972, Dr. Blackburn was appointed by the University of Minnesota to lead the Laboratory of Physiological Hygiene and later, its much larger descendant, the Division of Epidemiology and Community Health. Sometime around 1979 the direction of the Seven Countries Study was passed from Dr. Keys, who had officially retired in 1972 but still remained defacto leader, to the working group of Henry Blackburn, Dann Kromhout, then age 29, and Alessandro Menotti.[5] These three investigators worked closely together to keep the various parts of the Seven Countries Study together and, in some cases, to expand their scope. In the early 2000s, Dr. David Jacobs, a well-known epidemiologist and professor of Epidemiology at the University of Minnesota, joined the

3. Ibid., page 53.
4. Taylor HL, Klepetar E, Keys A, Parlin RW, Blackburn H, Puchner T. (1962) Death rates among physically active and sedentary employees of the railroad industry. *Am J Publ Health* 52: 1697-1707.
5. Personal communication from Dr. Henry Blackburn.

leadership team in order to provide advanced statistical analysis capability. The 25-year and 40-year follow-ups to the Seven Countries Study were spearheaded by Dr. Kromhout of the Netherlands and Dr. Menotti of Italy.

In 1999 the 25-year follow-up of the Seven Countries Study was published.[6] The 25-year coronary heart disease death rate in the men who were enrolled in the Seven Countries Study was, as in the previous updates, highest in East Finland and lowest in Crete, Greece. The next-highest death rates were in West Finland; then Zutphen, the Netherlands; and the fourth-highest was in the United Sates. After the data from Crete, the next lowest death rates were from the two cohorts in Japan. The full table from the article (Table 1) is shown below.

6. Alessandro Menotti, Daan Kromhout, Henry Blackburn, Flaminio Fidanza, Ratko Buzina, Aulikki Nissinens for the Seven Countries Study Research Group. (1999) Food intake patterns and 25-year mortality from coronary heart disease: Cross-cultural correlations in the Seven Countries Study. *European Journal of Epidemiology* 15: 507-515. http://www.ncbi.nlm.nih.gov/pubmed/?term=10485342

Table 1. Age-standardized 25-year death rates per 1000 from CHD in 16 cohorts of the Seven Countries Study. Standard error of rate in parenthesis

Cohorts	N	CHD (Death rates/1000)
US Railroad, USA	2571	160 (7)
East Finland, Finland	817	268 (15)
West Finland, Finland	860	180 (13)
Zutphen, The Netherlands	878	169 (13)
Crevalcore, Italy	993	93 (9)
Montegiorgio, Italy	719	60 (9)
Rome Railroad, Italy	768	87 (10)
Dalmatia, Croatia	671	54 (9)
Slavonia, Croatia	696	80 (10)
Velika Krsna, Serbia	511	43 (9)
Zrenjanin, Serbia	516	116 (14)
Belgrade, Serbia	536	106 (13)
Crete, Greece	686	25 (6)
Corfu, Greece	529	48 (9)
Tanushimaru, Japan	508	30 (8)
Ushibuka, Japan	502	36 (8)

From Menotti et al., (1999) *European Journal of Epidemiology* 15: 507-515. http://www.ncbi.nlm.nih.gov/pubmed/?term=10485342

The results from the analysis concerning food intake were succinctly described in the discussion of the paper:

> In fact, food patterns associated with high coronary heart disease mortality rates were characterized by high consumption of butter, dairy products and other animal products usually rich in saturated fatty acids and cholesterol. Food patterns associated with low or relatively low mortality rates from coronary heart disease were those

> characterized by high consumption of cereals, legumes, vegetable products, fish, oils and wine.[7]

The 40-year follow-up to the Seven Countries Study was published in 2007[8] and it is quite amazing that the participants in this study were in the age range 80 to 99 years old. Because the men were getting so old, they were starting to die of diseases associated with extreme aging. This is exemplified in the table of death rates shown below (Table 1 from the article), where the total death rates from the cohorts were approaching the maximal rate. However, when the coronary heart disease data from the entire 40 years of the study were analyzed together using the Weibull hazard rate (a statistical method for analyzing death data over a long period of time-see figure 2 from the article below), some interesting patterns were observed for some of the study cohorts. Serbia and Greece had upswings in their coronary heart disease death rates that mirrored the observations of Ancel and Margaret Keys that some countries were turning away from the Mediterranean diet because their socio-economic status increased or and some subindustrialized regions had merged their rural and urban areas. Finland and the United States tended to have lower rates further into the study as programs to alter fat intake and type took effect. The coronary heart disease rate in Japan remained consistently low, as one might expect, due to adherence of the Japanese to their low-fat diet. The 40-year follow-up report accentuated the concept that changing the diet could both lower and increase coronary heart disease death rates depending upon the nature of the changes made in the diet and the lifestyles of the participants.

7. Ibid., page 511.
8. Alessandro Menotti, Mariapaola Lanti, Daan Kromhout, Henry Blackburn, Aulikki Nissinen, Anastasios Dontas, Antony Kafatos, Srecko Nedeljkovic, Hisashi Adachi. (2007) Forty-year coronary mortality trends and changes in major risk factors in the first 10 years of follow-up in the seven countries study. *European Journal of Epidemiology* 22: 747–754. http://link.springer.com/article/10.1007%2Fs10654-007-9176-4

Table 1. Forty-year age adjusted death rates from coronary heart disease (CHD) and all causes in seven countries

Countries	N	CHD death rate per 1000 in 40 years		All causes death rate per 1000 in 40 years	
		Rate	s.e.	Rate	s.e.
United States	2,571	295	9	833	7
Finland	1,677	346	12	897	7
The Netherlands	878	260	15	874	11
Italy	1,712	165	9	826	9
Serbia	1,565	224	11	881	8
Greece	1,215	117	9	811	11
Japan	1,010	53	7	810	12

Table 1 from Menotti et al. (2007) *European Journal of Epidemiology* 22: 747–754. http://link.springer.com/article/10.1007%2Fs10654-007-9176-4

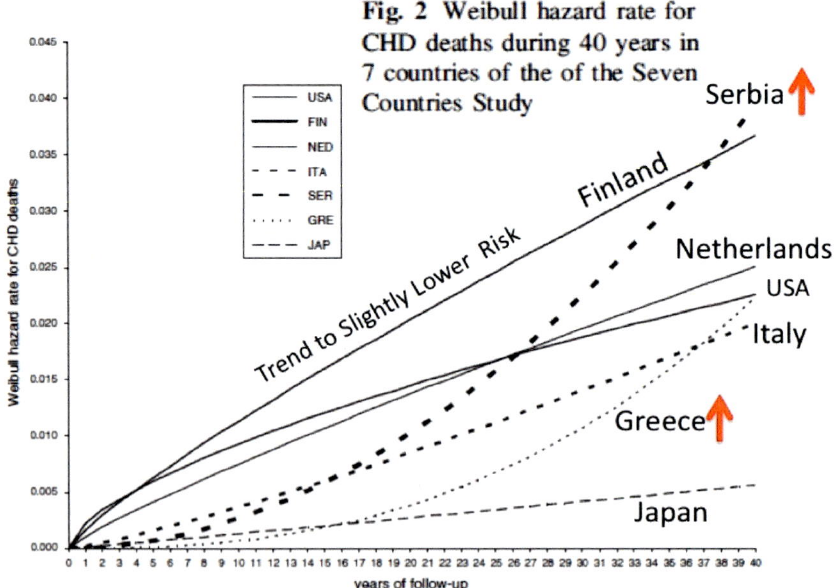

Figure 2 from Menotti et al. (2007) European Journal of Epidemiology.

The Seven Countries Study Continues to This Day!

Quite remarkably, the 50-year follow-up analysis is now complete[9] and contains data from all of the cohorts except those from Serbia, which is now unable to participate due to the destruction of the war in the 1990s. Drs. Alessandro Menotti and Daan Kromhout are still the main co-leaders of the Seven Countries Study. Dr. Henry Blackburn, with the assistance of the renowned epidemiologist, Dr. David Jacobs, still serves as an editor and advisor to the Seven Countries Study from the University of Minnesota. Also, quite remarkably, the Seven Countries Study has not received U.S. funding since 1979. The great majority of the funding for the study since then has come from the Netherlands and Italy.

At this point we will leave Ancel Keys, the Seven Countries Study, and the Mediterranean diet that was found to be protective against coronary heart disease. We will return to the story of Ancel and Margaret Keys after diving into the reasons for the existence of the mysterious molecule, cholesterol.

9. Personal communication from Dr. Henry Blackburn, August 2014.

PART II.

CHOLESTEROL: WHAT IS IT?

10.

DRS. GOLDSTEIN AND BROWN DISCOVER THE LDL RECEPTOR

Drs. Joseph Leonard Goldstein and Michael Stuart Brown giving their Nobel Prize Lectures at the Karolinska Institute, December 8, 1985

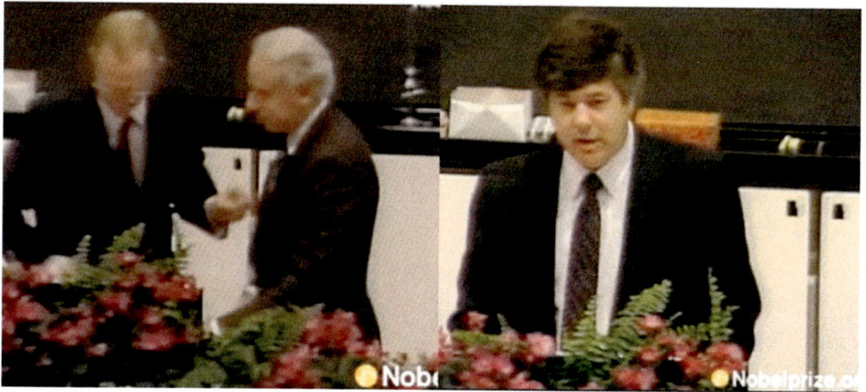

Screen shots of Drs. JL Goldstein (right in left panel) and MS Brown (right panel) delivering their 1985 Nobel Prize lectures. Permission received from the speakers and the Nobel Foundation.

When Ancel Keys and the Seven Countries Study researchers discovered that high cholesterol concentrations in blood were associated with coronary heart disease in middle-aged men, it highlighted the importance of this lipid that is actually found in fairly low concentration within cells. It was an established fact that cholesterol was a waxy substance, but there was very little known about it except that it was the starting material for a group of steroid hormones, including estrogen and testosterone.

Scientists were unaware of the function of cholesterol in the blood, nor how it was transported, until it was shown, by electrophoresis and ultracentrifugation, to be carried within lipoproteins in blood. The lipoprotein families were finally isolated and characterized in the late 1940s and early 1950s using several methods including the newly developed ultracentrifuge.

The slide below shows that most (about 75%) cholesterol in blood is carried within Low Density Lipoprotein (LDL). High density lipoprotein (HDL) also carries cholesterol in blood, but to a much lesser degree than LDL does. We will discuss HDL in a later chapter.

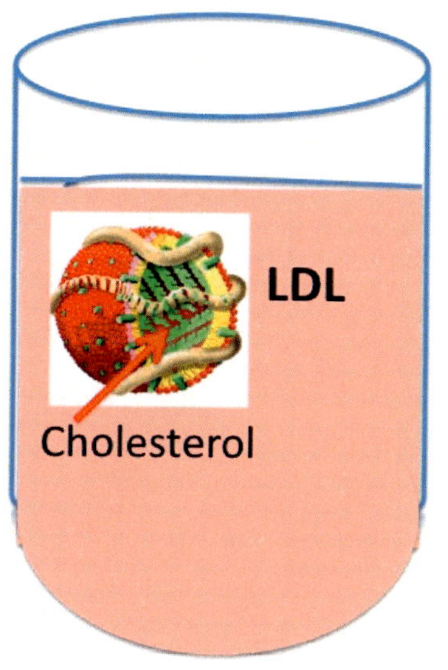

Most Cholesterol in Blood is Carried in Low Density Lipoprotein (LDL), a lipid droplet made up mostly of cholesteryl esters surrounded by a protein belt.

Most cholesterol (about 75%) in blood is carried within LDL, with the remaining being carried in other lipoprotein particles (not shown). Cholesterol is not present free in aqueous portion of blood to any major degree. Drawn by JL Dixon and J Byrd.

The following slide shows Very Low Density Lipoprotein (VLDL) (on left side) which primarily delivers fatty acids to cells, whereas LDL (on right side) delivers cholesterol (the multiring structure) to cells. VLDL is secreted by the liver and exists in blood for several hours until most of the triacylglycerol molecules it carries are hydrolyzed and the released fatty acids (drawn as a single long chain) are transferred to cells. After delivering fatty acids to cells, about 50% of VLDL is converted in blood to LDL, which mainly carries cholesterol in its core. LDL circulates in blood for several days and it mainly delivers cholesterol to cells, except for those in the brain, which LDL cannot enter due to the blood-brain barrier. The brain makes its own cholesterol.

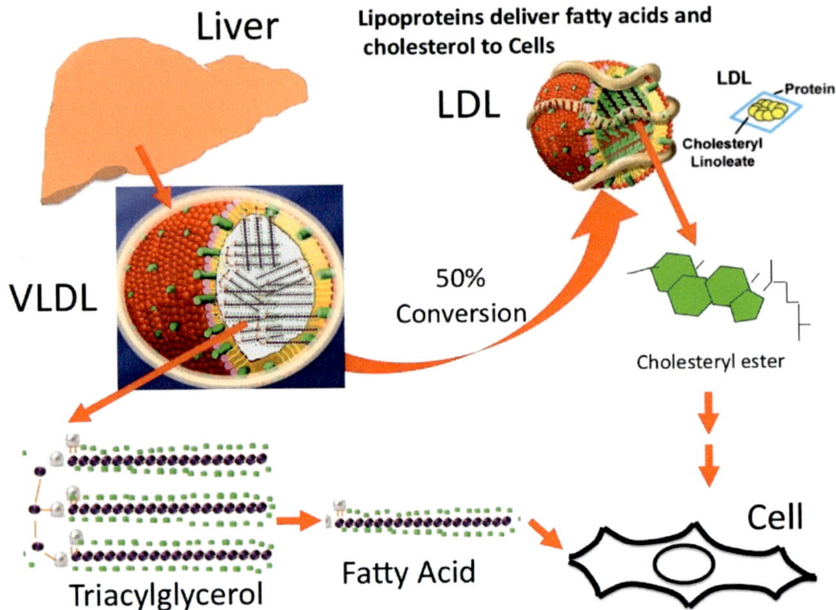

Functions of VLDL (left) and LDL (right) in blood. VLDL is secreted by liver cells and primarily carries triacylglycerol and delivers free fatty acids to peripheral cells, including heart muscle cells, immune cells, and finally, adipose cells. After considerable metabolism in blood, about 50% of VLDL is converted to LDL. LDL primarily carries cholesterol as cholesteryl esters and delivers cholesterol to peripheral cells. Drawn by JL Dixon.

Studies on the transport of fatty acids, cholesterol, and lipoproteins using radioisotopes and other methods continued through the 1950s and 1960s (Fredrickson 1958), but there was still uncertainty about how lipoprotein particles interacted with cells, and how cholesterol in the lipoproteins actually got into the cells.[1]

The mystery surrounding cholesterol and low density lipoprotein in blood persisted until two scientists unraveled the metabolism and function of the LDL receptor.[2] The story of these

1. Fredrickson DS, Gordon, Jr, RS. (1958) Transport of fatty acids. *Physiol. Rev.* 38: 585–630. http://physrev.physiology.org/content/38/4/585.long

two young assistant professors demonstrates the power of partnership in attaining extraordinary accomplishments.

Drs. Joseph Leonard Goldstein and Michael Stuart Brown met when they were interns at the Massachusetts General Hospital in Boston. Later on, they would reunite and work together on cholesterol metabolism at the University of Texas Southwestern Medical School in Dallas. Their experiences in various laboratories and medical centers during their training prepared them for tackling the biochemical mystery of what controlled blood cholesterol levels.[3]

Dr. Goldstein was born in South Carolina in 1940 and went to college at Washington and Lee University in Lexington, Virginia. After medical school in Dallas at the Southwestern Medical School, he interned in Boston and then worked at the National Heart Institute in Bethesda, Maryland. One of his supervisors at the NIH was Dr. Marshall W. Nirenberg, who would later share the Nobel Prize in Medicine and Physiology for deciphering the genetic code. Dr. Goldstein then spent two years working at the University of Washington in Seattle studying why patients suffered heart attacks. He focused on the complicated genetics that were responsible for certain forms of hyperlipidemias. With these experiences, Dr. Goldstein returned to the Southwestern Medical School as a faculty member.

Dr. Brown is a native of New York City and was born in 1941. He obtained undergraduate and medical degrees from the University of Pennsylvania in Philadelphia. After he interned in Boston and met Dr. Goldstein, he worked at the National Institutes of Health in the Digestive and Hereditary Disease Branch, where he studied enzymes involved in digestion. He moved to the University of

2. Goldstein JL, Brown MS. (2009) The LDL receptor. *Arterioscler Thromb Vasc Biol.* 29(4): 431-438. http://atvb.ahajournals.org/content/29/4/431.long
3. Sullivan, Walter. (1985) Men in the news: Dr. Joseph L. Goldstein and Dr. Michael S. Brown; converging on a Nobel prize. *New York Times*, October 15, 1985. http://www.nytimes.com/1985/10/15/science/men-dr-joseph-l-goldstein-dr-michael-s-brown-converging-nobel-prize.html

Texas Southwestern Medical School and began studying enzymes involved in cholesterol metabolism. In 1971 he reunited with Dr. Goldstein to study the disease, hypercholesterolemia (high blood cholesterol), and their collaboration eventually led to the discovery of the LDL receptor.

The road to the Nobel Prize began when Drs. Brown and Goldstein sought the metabolic reason for familial hypercholesterolemia (FH), a genetic disease where the concentration of cholesterol in blood is increased enormously compared to healthy controls, and where cholesterol deposits, called xanthomas, appear in the skin. These patients have heart attacks early in life, sometimes as early as 6 years old.

Drs. Goldstein and Brown cultured skin cells from patients who had familial hypercholesterolemia (FH), and compared cholesterol metabolism in them with its metabolism in fibroblasts from normal patients. They showed that adding very low concentrations of LDL to normal cultured fibroblasts lowered the cells' activity of hydroxy methylglutaryl Coenzyme A reductase, a key enzyme in cholesterol synthesis. This experimental result pointed to the fact that when added to the outside of cells, LDL could affect cholesterol metabolism within the cells.

Surprisingly, fibroblasts from FH patients did not react to treatment with LDL, so something was wrong with the ability of these cells to use LDL. Eventually, Drs. Goldstein and Brown determined that FH fibroblasts have a defective protein called the LDL receptor, which was involved in bringing LDL from blood into the interior of cells. Cholesterol delivered to the cell with LDL is delivered using the LDL receptor, a protein that is located on the plasma membrane surface of all cells. Once cholesterol enters the cell, it is capable of affecting (in this case, feedback regulating) cholesterol metabolism within the cell.

After purifying the LDL receptor protein, the laboratories of Drs. Goldstein and Brown went on to clone the gene for the LDL receptor, and show that the molecular defect in FH was a mutation in the LDL receptor protein.

Then commenced a series of studies investigating the LDL receptor and how it works. Cell biology studies showed that LDL receptors were either degraded in the lysosome or recycled to the cell membrane.[4] It turned out that the LDL receptor was used over and over again to bring LDL lipoproteins into cells. After the receptor picked up LDL, it carried it into the cell, released it, and then traveled back to the membrane to start the process all over again. At some point an LDL receptor was marked for degradation in the lysosome.

To discover the actual mechanism of LDL uptake, Drs. Brown and Goldstein collaborated with a cell biologist, Richard G.W. Anderson, who happened to be located in the same building at the University of Texas Southwestern Medical Center in Dallas. This is an example of the apparent likelihood that fortuitous circumstances are often involved in scientific discovery. Dr. Anderson studied LDL receptors by following the uptake of LDL (coupled to electron-dense ferritin) into cells using the electron microscope. The figure below shows how LDL molecules attached to LDL receptors first cluster on the surface of cells in "coated pits," that then "pinch off from the surface to form coated endocytic vesicles that carry extracellular fluid and its contents into the cell."[5] [6] These magnificent images of LDL being taken up into cells gave strength to the assertions of Drs. Brown and

4. Goldstein JL, Brunschede GY, Brown MS. (1975) Inhibition of the proteolytic degradation of low density lipoprotein in human fibroblasts by chloroquine, concanavalinA, and Triton WR1339. *J Biol Chem* 250: 7854–7862. http://www.jbc.org/content/250/19/7854.long
5. Anderson RGW, Brown MS, Goldstein JL. (1977) Role of the coated endocytic vesicle in the uptake of receptor-bound low density lipoprotein in human fibroblasts. *Cell* 10: 351–364. http://www.ncbi.nlm.nih.gov/pubmed/?term=Cell.+1977+Mar%3B10%283%29%3A351-64
6. Brown MS, Goldstein JL. (2011) Richard G.W. Anderson (1940-2011) and the birth of receptor-mediated endocytosis. *J Cell Biol* 193(4): 601-603. http://jcb.rupress.org/content/193/4/601.long

Goldstein that what they were studying was a real biological phenomenon. Of course, Drs. Brown and Goldstein, through biochemical experiments, would later confirm the mechanism suggested by these photographs.

Richard G.W. Anderson's first sighting of LDL receptors in human fibroblasts.

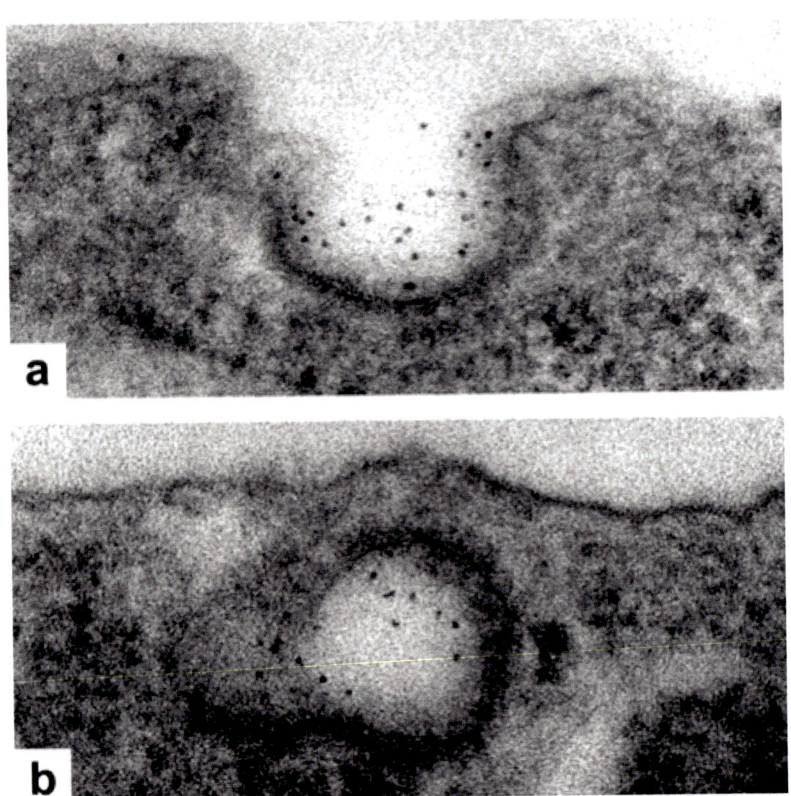

Brown MS, Goldstein JL. (2011) *J Cell Biol* 193: 601-603.
Anderson RGW, Brown MS, Goldstein JL. (1977) Cell 10: 351–364.

LDL receptors visualized using LDL-ferritin (black dots) in so-called "coated pits" on the surface of a cell (a) and inside the cell (b). RGW Anderson captured these electron micrographs of human fibroblasts in 1975 and they were republished in 2011 (©2011 Brown and Goldstein. Journal of Cell Biology. 193:601-603. doi:10.1083/jcb.201104136).

Subsequently, Drs. Goldstein and Brown went on to delineate in fine detail the exact mechanism of uptake of LDL into cells via the LDL receptor, and how the delivery of cholesterol to cells in LDL can modulate multiple pathways that control cholesterol metabolism within cells. This is diagrammed on the fairly complex figure below that was in the cited review article by Drs. Goldstein and Brown.[7] I have placed the images of Drs. Anderson, Goldstein, and Brown over the diagram so that the original observations and the drawn representations are displayed in juxtaposition.

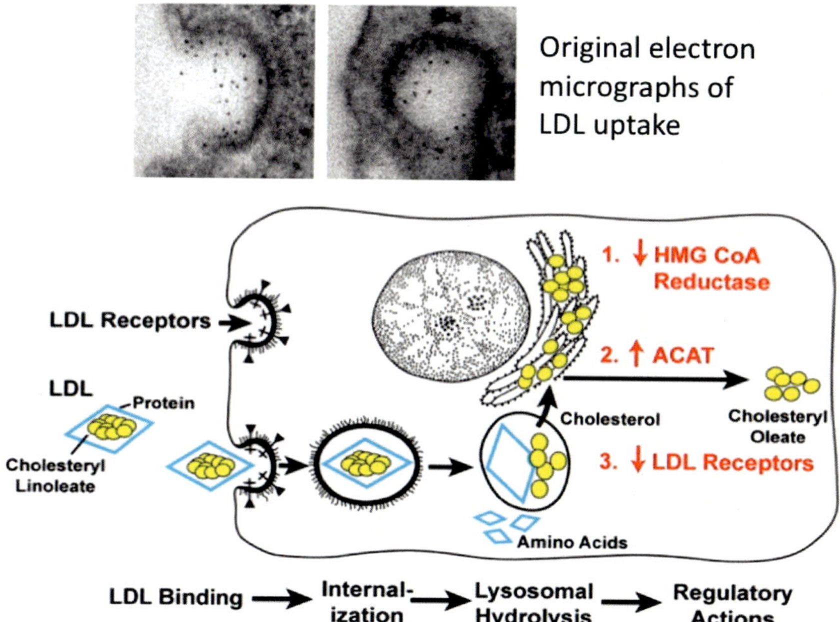

The top image is from Brown MS, Goldstein JL (©2011 Brown and Goldstein. *Journal of Cell Biology*. 193:601-603. doi:10.1083/jcb.201104136). The lower diagram showing the sequential step in the LDL receptor pathway in animal cells is from Goldstein JL, Brown MS. (2009) *Arterioscler Thromb Vasc Biol* 29: 431-438.

7. Goldstein JL, Brown MS. (2009) The LDL receptor. *Arterioscler Thromb Vasc Biol*. 29(4): 431-438. http://atvb.ahajournals.org/content/29/4/431.long

The red text within the cell diagram lists the major effects that occur in metabolism when LDL cholesterol was experimentally delivered to cells. First (see #1 inside the cell), the activity of hydroxymethyl glutaryl coenzyme A reductase (HMG CoA reductase), an important regulatory enzyme in cholesterol synthesis, is decreased. Second, cholesterol esterification is increased in order to store extra cholesterol as cholesteryl esters in the cell's lipid droplets. Third, the numbers of LDL receptor protein molecules on the cell's membrane are decreased in order to slow the influx of cholesterol into the cell through the LDL receptor uptake pathway.

The discovery of the LDL receptor gave rise to a wide new avenue of research in cell biology that helped scientists understand how cells work. Not only did the discovery of the LDL receptor provide insights into how lipoproteins are taken up by cells, but it gave rise to the eventual discovery of many other receptors and complex receptor-mediated uptake mechanisms used by all cells. For this major discovery, Drs. Goldstein and Brown won the Nobel Prize in Physiology or Medicine on October 15, 1985 (see their picture taken on this day below; their lectures can be watched on the Nobel prize website).[8] [9]

8. http://www.nobelprize.org/nobel_prizes/medicine/laureates/1985/goldstein-lecture.html
9. http://www.nobelprize.org/nobel_prizes/medicine/laureates/1985/brown-lecture.html

Figure 6. Joseph L. Goldstein (left) and Michael S. Brown on the day of announcement of their Nobel Prize in Physiology or Medicine on October 15, 1985.

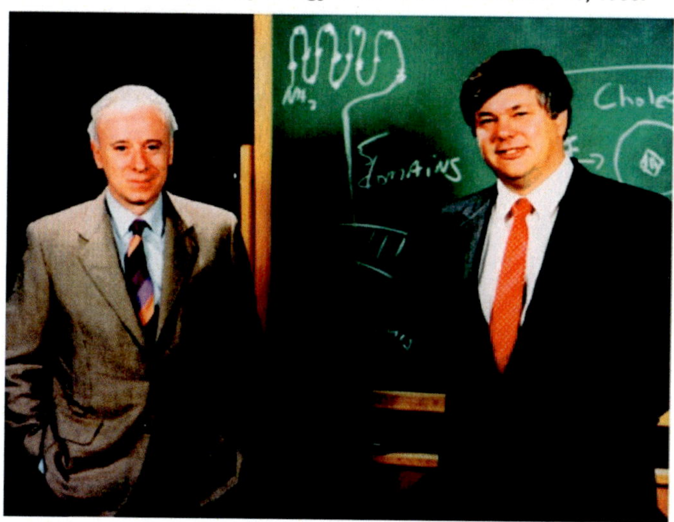

Goldstein J L , and Brown M S Arterioscler Thromb Vasc Biol. 2009;29:431-438

Drs. Goldstein and Brown would go on to make many more amazing discoveries in cellular cholesterol and lipid metabolism. These additional discoveries include deciphering: 1) the complex mechanism of sterol receptor element binding proteins (SREBPs), proteins that direct the transcription of genes involved in both cholesterol and fatty acid metabolism; 2) the cholesterol sensor in the membrane of the endoplasmic reticulum; and 3) several transport mechanisms used to move cholesterol throughout the cell. Furthermore, Drs. Goldstein and Brown have made many contributions to the understanding of numerous human disease states that involve lipid metabolism, including several hyperlipidemias, the metabolic syndrome, and type 2 diabetes. Many researchers throughout biochemistry, and especially in the lipid field, strongly believe that Drs. Goldstein and Brown deserve to be awarded a second Nobel Prize in medicine. I personally endorse this as well! The collaboration between Dr. Goldstein and Dr. Brown continues to this day.[10]

10. http://www4.utsouthwestern.edu/moleculargenetics/pages/gold/lab.html

11.

WHY IS THERE CHOLESTEROL IN THE BODY?

There is no other molecule that instills more anxiety in humans than cholesterol. Go to the doctor and if he or she tells you that your blood cholesterol is too high, you will begin to worry about your health and the possibility of future problems with heart disease.

While teaching my class in nutrition and health over the past twenty-five years, I have attempted to give a more balanced view of cholesterol and the only way to do this is to explain what cholesterol does in the body. I do this by comparing plant cells and human cells. Plant cells do not contain cholesterol. Plant cells have a membrane that surrounds every cell, but in addition, plant cells have an exterior cell wall that is thicker than the cell membrane underneath it. Human cells do not have a cell wall, and therefore, their cell membranes need to be strengthened in another way. The way mammalian cells strengthen their membranes is to insert cholesterol into them. The slide below shows how I envision the role cholesterol plays as a structural molecule. Cholesterol has four rings that can be stacked on top of each other in the membrane, just like a common building material, the cinder block! Not only do cholesterol molecules act like a single cinder block, but they act like side by side cinder blocks, which provide more strength. The next slide shows cholesterol situated in the membrane. When cholesterol is in the membrane, it promotes organization, anchors other lipids, and strengthens the bilayer of phospholipids that line up and form the membrane.

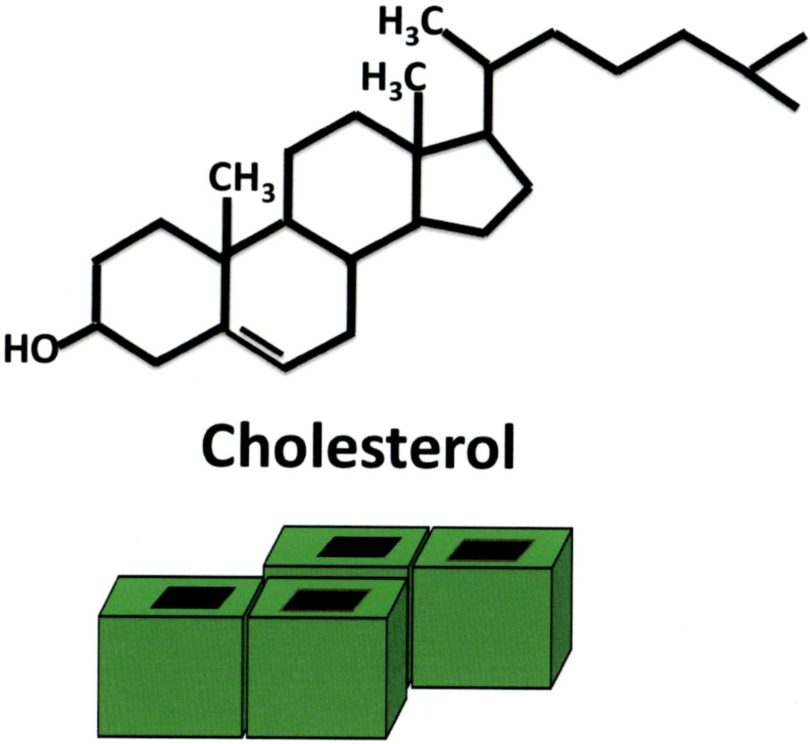

Cholesterol

The cholesterol molecule can be considered a biological cinder block that can provide strength and rigidity to the plasma membrane. The green cinder block representation is used in the next series of drawings. Drawing by JL Dixon.

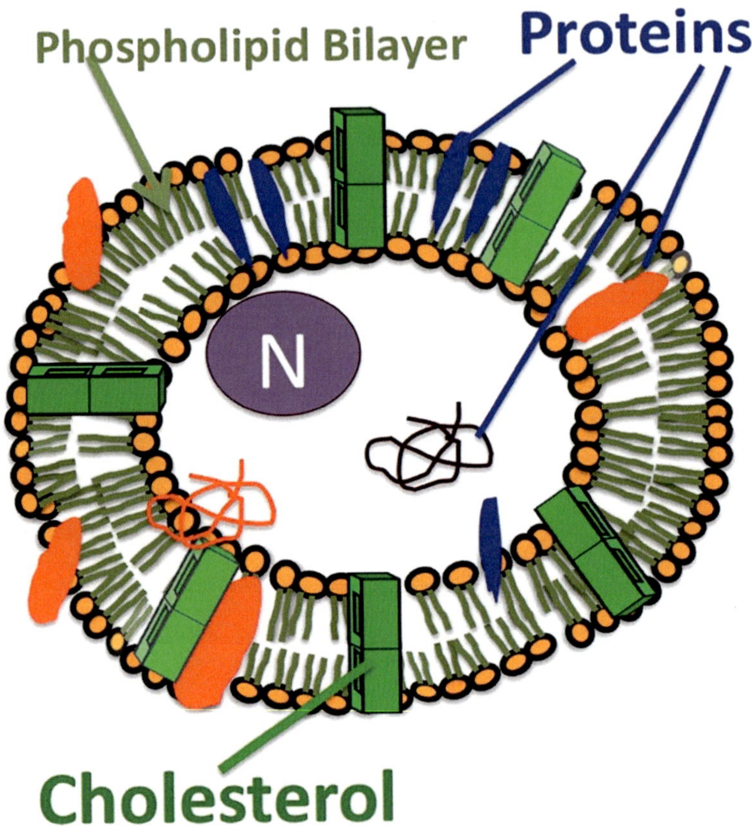

Cholesterol strengthens the plasma membrane in animal cells. The image shows the membrane portion of the cell without internal structures depicted except for the nucleus (N). The cholesterol molecule in the membrane is represented by a green cinder block. Drawing by JL Dixon.

The image below (which is the starting image of an eight hour time lapsed movie of a live cell) shows the distribution of free cholesterol in live HeLa cells in culture. HeLa cells are immortal human cells that can grow in culture and derive from a biopsy from Henritta Lacks.[1] HeLa cells are often used to study basic aspects of cell growth and function. In order to visual cholesterol in cells, we added cholesterol molecules that have a fluorescent marker attached (BODIPY-cholesterol, shows green in the image) and examined the cells with a microscope in order to determine where the green traveled to in the live cells. In this first image of the movie, most of the green is seen in the membrane, and this indicates that a majority of free cholesterol is localized in the membrane. Green is also seen in lipid droplets that show up as circles in the interior of the cell. This image of a live cell shows that free cholesterol is, indeed, concentrated in the cell membrane where it adds strength and structure to the membrane.[2]

1. Skloot, Rebecca (2010) *The Immortal Life of Henrietta Lacks*. New York: Crown Publishing (Random House).
2. Ilnytska O, Santiana M, Hsu NY, Du WL, Chen YH, Viktorova EG, Belov G, Brinker A, Storch J, Moore C, Dixon JL, Altan-Bonnet N. (2013) Enteroviruses harness the cellular endocytic machinery to remodel the host cell cholesterol landscape for effective viral replication. *Cell Host and Microbe*. 14(3): 281-293. http://www.sciencedirect.com/science/article/pii/S1931312813002667

Movie S1_1: BODIPY-cholesterol (green) dynamics in HeLa cells

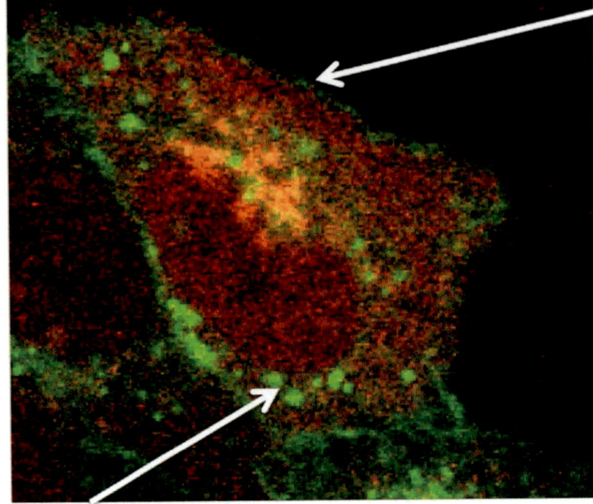

Live HeLA cell showing the normal locations of free cholesterol within the cell. The green in the membrane and in the small round droplets is fluorescence from BODIPY-cholesterol. The image is a frame from a movie taken of a live cell. From Ilnytska et al. (2013) *Cell Host and Microbe* 14(3): 281-293.

As with any component of the cell, precise roles played by cholesterol are not easily discerned. Early studies showed that cholesterol in the membrane prevents movement of the fatty acyl chains of phospholipids in the membrane, a process that is called fluidity.[3] When phospholipids are held in place, the membrane is more rigid and stronger.

Much of the laboratory work on the role of cholesterol content on membrane function was performed in the 1960s and 1970s

3. Spector AA, Yorek MA. (1985) Membrane lipid composition and cellular function. *J Lipid Res.* 26(9): 1015-1035. http://www.jlr.org/content/26/9/1015.long

and was concisely reviewed in a chapter in John Sabine's book, *Cholesterol.*[4]

In the red blood cell membrane, there are approximately 0.9 cholesterol molecules for every phospholipid molecule. In other types of cells, the composition ranges from 0.25 to 0.5 cholesterol molecules per phospholipid molecule.[5] However, in the brain, the myelin sheath that surrounds nerve cells is especially rich in cholesterol as it contains about 1.3 molecules of cholesterol per phospholipid molecule.[6] This means that there are more than twice as many cholesterol molecules relative to phosphoslipid molecules in myelin compared to the membranes of most other cells.

The ability of small molecules to travel through the membrane is affected by the amount of cholesterol in the plasma membrane. The greater the amount of cholesterol in a membrane, the less water, glucose, glycerol, sodium, choride, and other small molecules that can diffuse through the membrane.[7] Additionally, cholesterol in the membrane allows certain proteins in the membrane to function properly.[8] In general, cholesterol makes the plasma membrane of cells less fragile and allows the membrane to work properly for that particular kind of cell.

The cholesterol molecule emerged early in evolution and because of its properties, it was used by early organisms for other purposes besides making the membrane stronger. One of the other purposes of cholesterol is to supply the starting molecule for the synthesis of the steroid hormones. Therefore, testosterone, estrogen, cortisol, progesterone, vitamin D, and other steroid hormones are all made from cholesterol.

4. Sabine JR. (1977) "The role of cholesterol in membrane systems," in *Cholesterol*, New York: Marcel Dekker.
5. Ibid., page 10.
6. Ibid., page 10.
7. Ibid., page 19.
8. Farías RN, Bloj B, Morero RD, Siñeriz F, Trucco RE. (1975) Regulation of allosteric membrane-bound enzymes through changes in membrane lipid composition. *Biochimica et Biophysica Acta* 415(2):231-251.

Another major function of cholesterol in the body is that it is used in the synthesis of the bile salts, which are secreted into the lumen of the intestine to solubilize lipids from foods. Without bile salts the efficiency of the uptake of dietary lipids from the intestinal lumen would be greatly reduced. An additional function is that cholesterol is required for neuron function and the process of learning and the establishment of memory.

Almost every cell in the body has the ability to make cholesterol from the very basic, two-carbon acetate molecule. The synthesis of cholesterol, and many of the enzymes required, were elucidated in the 1950s in several laboratories, including the laboratory of Konrad Bloch, who received the Nobel Prize in Physiology or Medicine in 1964. This prize was awarded jointly to Dr. Bloch and Dr. Feodor Lynen "for their discoveries concerning the mechanism and regulation of the cholesterol and fatty acid metabolism." The most amazing reactions of the long synthetic pathway for cholesterol are the folding and cyclization of the intermediate, squalene, to form lanosterol, which is a four ring structure.[9] The body goes to great lengths to synthesize cholesterol in every cell. From these observations, it is clear that cholesterol plays several important roles in the body and we would not be able to survive without it.

How much cholesterol is in the body?

A 70 kg male has about 140 g of cholesterol in his entire body of which 32 g (22%) are in the brain and nerves; 22% is in adipose, connective tissue, and fluids other than blood; 21% is in the muscle; and the remaining 35% is distributed throughout the other tissues.[10] To put the amount of cholesterol that is

9. Tchen TT, Bloch K. (1957) On the mechanism of enzymatic cyclization of squalene. *J Biol Chem* 226(2): 931-939. http://www.jbc.org/content/226/2/931.long
10. Cook, Robert P. (Editor) (1958) *Cholesterol: Chemistry, Biochemistry, and Pathology*. New York: Academic Press Inc. Values from Chapter 4 by Robert P.

consumed in the diet into perspective, most Americans consume 100 to 500 mg of cholesterol per day. An intake of 200 mg represents 0.2g/140g of the cholesterol in the body; this dietary cholesterol represents 0.14% of the cholesterol in the body of a 70 kg male. A comparison of the amount of cholesterol consumed per day by humans to the amount of cholesterol that is already in the body is depicted in the following figure:

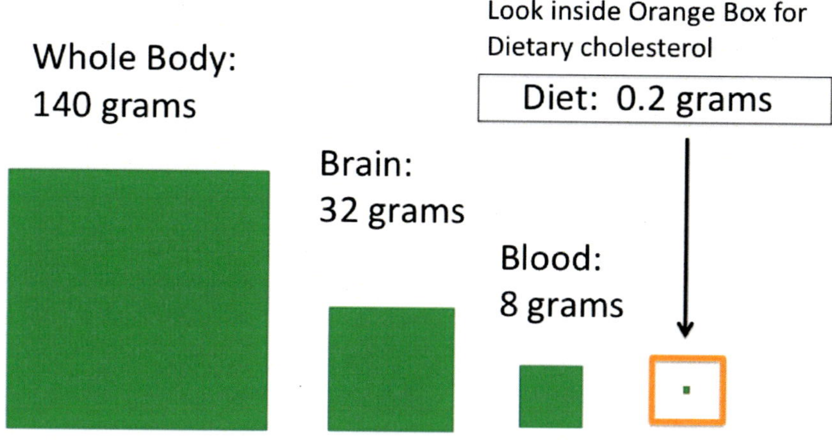

Amount of cholesterol consumed in the diet is small compared to the total amount of cholesterol in the body. Data from Robert Cook (1958), page 174. Figure by JL Dixon.

If cholesterol is a such an important and necessary molecule, why is it so bad for us?

Cholesterol is bad for us when it builds up in the wrong places.

Cook, "Distribution of Sterols in Organisms and in Tissues," Table XVI, page 174.

One of those places is the blood where cholesterol is carried mostly in Low Density Lipoprotein (LDL) particles.

What is LDL? Since cholesterol is a lipid (a fatty substance) and blood is mostly water, and oil and water don't mix, there has to be a special way of transporting cholesterol through the blood. LDL (see image below) is a lipid droplet surrounded by a large, structural, belt-like protein called apolipoprotein B (or ApoB for short).[11] The lipid droplet of LDL has a surrounding phospholipid layer that also has an occasional free cholesterol molecule inserted in it. The core of the particle is made of approximately 1,500 cholesteryl ester molecules in a semicrystalline packing. Cholesteryl esters are cholesterol molecules with a fatty acid (usually oleic acid) attached to one end. The close-up image shows how the phospholipid (in the box) orientates in the surface covering with its two fatty acids (yellow legs) facing in and the positively charged head group (usually a choline molecule, depicted in red) facing outward toward the water of blood. This lipoprotein structure allows for the solubility of the cholesterol in blood and its transport throughout the body.

11. Richardson MR, Lai X, Dixon JL, Sturek M, Witzmann FA. (2009) Diabetic dyslipidemia and exercise alter the plasma low-density lipoproteome in Yucatan pigs. *Proteomics* 9(9): 2468-2483. http://www.ncbi.nlm.nih.gov/pmc/articles/PMC2859442/

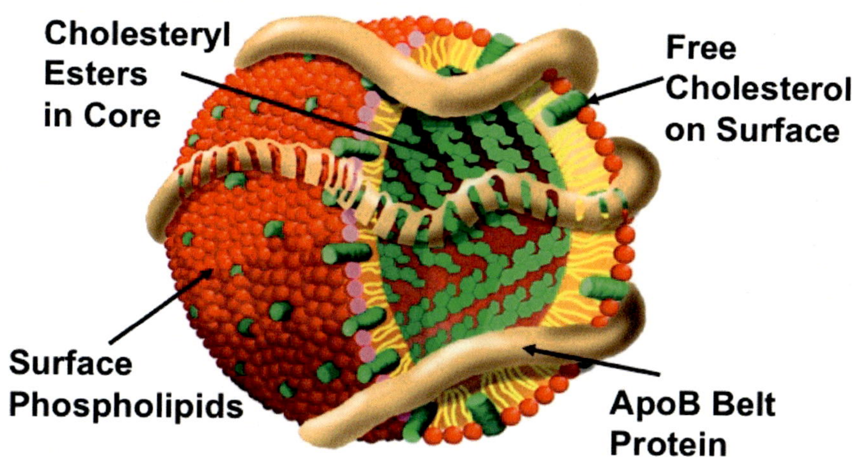

Drawing of Low Density Lipoprotein (LDL). LDL is a lipid particle surrounded by a large structural protein called apolipoprotein B (ApoB). The lipid portion is made of surface phospholipids (red and yellow) and a small number of cholesterol molecules (green barrels). The interior is mostly cholesteryl esters (ring structures) and a small amount of triglyceride (not shown). Drawing by J. Dixon and J. Byrd. A version of this figure was used in Richardson et al. (2009) *Proteomics* 9(9): 2468-2483. http://www.ncbi.nlm.nih.gov/pmc/articles/PMC2859442/

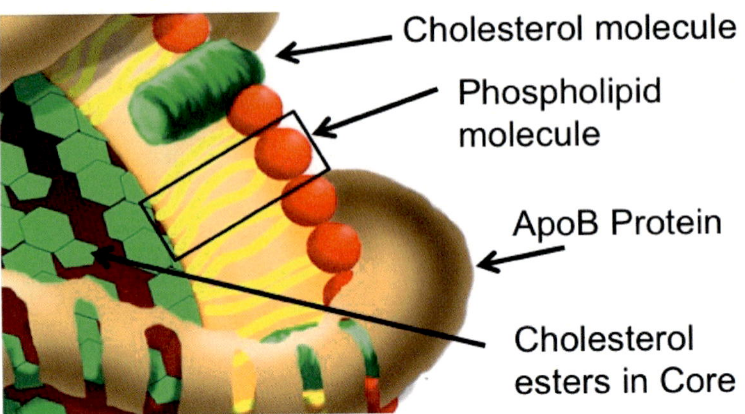

Drawing by J Dixon and J Byrd

For most of us, for most of our lives, there is no problem with cholesterol in the blood. But with age the number of LDL receptors on the surface of cells naturally declines (like many other functions that decline with age), and therefore, the LDL concentration builds up in blood. With increased LDL in blood, over time the LDL particles can enter the artery wall and start to build up within the wall. Therefore, cholesterol also builds up within the artery wall and can become so concentrated that cholesterol crystals begin to form. At some point this becomes severe, and with the occurrence of several other events, may cause the blockage of the major conduit arteries (coronary arteries) in the heart, causing a heart attack.

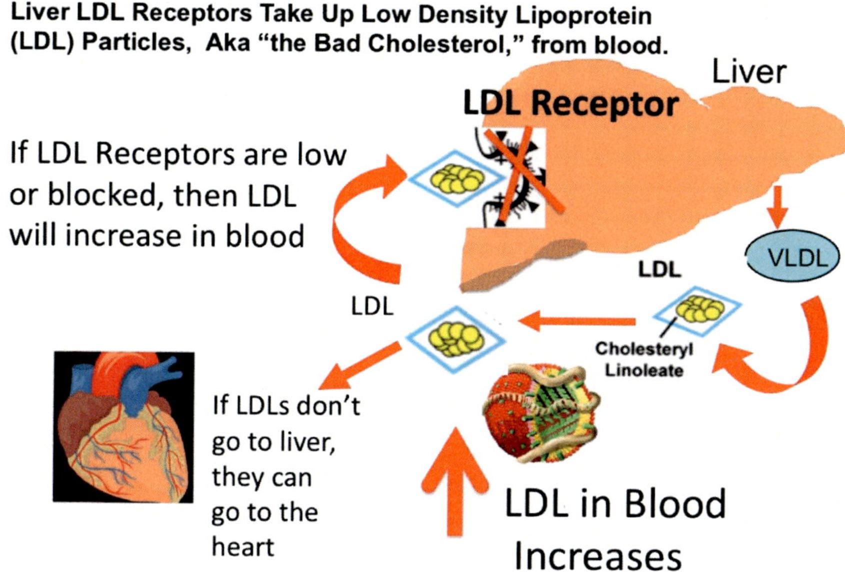

Diagram explaining how LDL increases with age. VLDL is secreted by liver cells and about 50% is converted to LDL in blood. The diamonds with yellow circles and the red-yellow-green ball represent LDL molecules. The red X indicates that there are lower LDL receptors on the membranes of liver cells as humans age. The diamonds and LDL receptors are depictions used previously by Drs. Goldstein and Brown. If LDL builds up in the blood, it has a greater propensity to enter the artery walls in the heart. Drawing by JL Dixon.

So for the most part, the system that controls cholesterol in the body works fine until we start to get into our 50s or older. Remember, up until recently, most humans did not live longer than 50 years of age. Therefore, having the cholesterol regulatory system break down after age 50 had only minimal effects on human evolution and survival. Of course, with the consumption of certain diets, the blood cholesterol can be driven higher, and then problems with cholesterol regulation occur much earlier than age 50. Also, as was observed in patients who had familial hypercholesterolemia (FH), or in patients with other hyperlipidemias, the system that controls cholesterol can be genetically disturbed and cause heart attacks even in young humans.

How does diet affect the cholesterol regulatory system in humans? How does high LDL cause the blockage of arteries?

These are extremely complex questions and they are still controversial. The studies of Dr. Ancel Keys of the University of Minnesota and other researchers showed that dietary saturated fat increased blood cholesterol concentrations. The exact molecular mechanism how this occurs is not known. We will put this discussion off until we discuss statins in chapter 12.

To be honest, the precise structure of cholesterol in membranes is still being studied and debated. For example, cholesterol and sphingomyelin are closely associated and form 1:1 dimers in the membrane. Also, the membrane contains different regions of organization and cholesterol is required to form specific distinct regions. Cholesterol is crucial to the formation of the correct orientation of certain membrane proteins in the membrane by providing hydrophobic regions and changing the membrane thickness in certain regions. A recent review of this topic has just been published.[12]

Cholesterol in the Brain

The human brain contains about 25% of the body's total cholesterol, and a large amount of the brain cholesterol, and possibly all of it, is synthesized in the brain.[13] In the past several

12. Nicolson GL (2014) The Fluid—Mosaic Model of Membrane Structure: Still relevant to understanding the structure, function and dynamics of biological membranes after more than 40 years. *Biochimica et Biophysica Acta* 1838: 1451–1466. http://www.sciencedirect.com/science/article/pii/S0005273613003933
13. Dietschy JM, Turley SD. (2004) Thematic review series: brain Lipids. Cholesterol metabolism in the central nervous system during early

years, studies have provided evidence that dysfunctional cholesterol metabolism in the brain may be involved in Huntington's disease. Neurons themselves have low rates of cholesterol synthesis, and they obtain most of their cholesterol from nearby helper cells called astrocytes (See figure below). The cholesterol made in the astrocyte needs to be shuttled to the neuron by lipoproteins containing apolipoprotein E (ApoE). ApoE is another protein that is used to form lipoproteins. Without adequate cholesterol, proper myelin and new nerve connections cannot be formed during the learning process. In a review of the role of cholesterol in Huntington's Disease (HD),[14] the authors stated,

> Although additional research is needed, molecular and biochemical studies in cellular and animal models of HD and in tissue and fluid samples from HD patients indicate that cholesterol biosynthesis is affected in HD. Data from multiple rodent models support the hypothesis that reduced activity of the cholesterol biosynthetic pathway and lower brain cholesterol levels are associated with HD, which suggests that enhancement of brain cholesterol biosynthesis and/or availability might ameliorate aspects of this disease.

The roles of cholesterol in the brain, and in other brain conditions such as Alzheimer's disease, are just beginning to be studied in great detail. In fact, there are still methodological problems measuring cholesterol in the brain. The figure below is from the review by Drs. Valenza and Cattaneo concerning Huntington's disease.[15]

development and in the mature animal. *J Lipid Res* 45, 1375–1397. http://www.jlr.org/content/45/8/1375.long

14. Valenza M, Cattaneo E. (2011) Emerging roles for cholesterol in Huntington's disease. *Trends in Neurosciences* 34(9): 474-486. http://www.sciencedirect.com/science/article/pii/S0166223611000932
15. Ibid., page 481

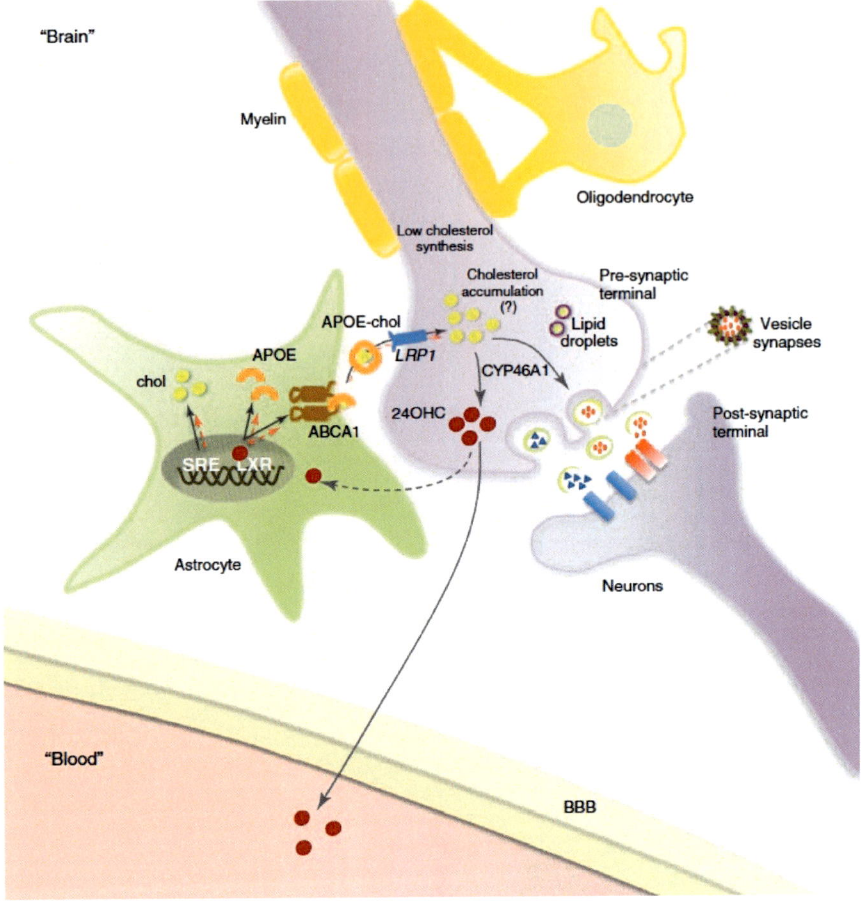

Cholesterol Metabolism in Brain. Cholesterol is synthesized in the astrocyte and transferred to the neuron on apoE-lipoproteins. Cholesterol is highly concentrated in the myelin regions of the neuronal membrane. Cholesterol is also metabolized (Red balls labeled 24OHC) and released into the blood. From Valenza M, Cattaneo E. (2011) *Trends in Neurosciences* 34(9): 474-486.

Cholesterol Is Involved in Memory

The effects of blood cholesterol levels, and in particular, the serum LDL-cholesterol concentration, on memory and learning have been studied[16] and there appears to be no concrete data indicating that there is a connection between these parameters. Because LDL doesn't cross the blood brain barrier this observation makes physiological sense.

But studies have indicated that the cholesterol made in the brain is involved in memory. Spatial learning, associative learning, and motor learning were all decreased in mice with a deficiency of cholesterol 24-hydroxylase, indicating a role for an enzyme involved in cholesterol turnover in memory or learning.[17] Mice that lacked the cholesterol 24-hydroxylase enzyme in brain had normal concentrations of cholesterol in the brain, but cholesterol synthesis in brain was reduced by about 40%. Apparently, loss of this enzyme involved in the turnover of cholesterol resulted in decreased synthesis of cholesterol due to a feedback regulation mechanism. Addition of 0.2 mM geranylgeraniol, a metabolite in the cholesterol synthesis pathway, restored some aspects of the metabolic defect when tested in slices of brain tissue. The exact function of geranylgeraniol is not known, but it may act as a signaling molecule at the membrane surface. Also, one can't rule out that newly synthesized cholesterol is used for specialized membrane synthesis during learning. This may have been one of the deficiencies in the mice with the cholesterol 24-hydroxylase enzyme knocked out. These studies support the need for very high amounts of cholesterol synthesis in the brain in order to maintain normal learning.

16. Schreurs BG. (2010) The effects of cholesterol on learning and memory, *Neuroscience and Biobehavioral Reviews* 34: 1366–1379 http://www.sciencedirect.com/science/article/pii/S0149763410000941
17. Kotti TJ, Ramirez DMO, Pfeiffer BE, Huber KM, Russell DW. (2006) Brain cholesterol turnover required for geranylgeraniol production and learning in mice. *Proc Natl Acad Sci U.S.A.* 103: 3869–3874. http://www.pnas.org/content/103/10/3869.long

One thing is for certain: No cholesterol synthesis — No new neurons — No learning![18]

18. Russell DW, Halford RW, Ramirez DM, Shah R, Kotti T. (2009) Cholesterol 24-hydroxylase: an enzyme of cholesterol turnover in the brain. *Annu Rev Biochem* 78: 1017-1040. http://www.ncbi.nlm.nih.gov/pubmed/?term=19489738

12.

THE FRAMINGHAM STUDY, THE MOUNT EVEREST OF EPIDEMIOLOGICAL STUDIES

Whereas the Seven Countries Study was an ecological, epidemiological study that was carried out across a wide range of countries, climates, cultures, and culinary customs, the Framingham study was an epidemiological study supported by the National Heart Institute (the forerunner of the National Heart, Lung, and Blood Institute) that was planned to be carried out in a single location with participants having a fairly focused genetic background and a fairly uniform diet (i.e., the American diet at the time).

In addition to Dr. Ancel Keys's Seven Countries Study, much of what we know about risk factors for coronary heart disease have come, first and foremost, from the Framingham Study and cohort studies that followed it and confirmed it in other populations. When Ancel Keys published his 15-year follow-up study on coronary heart disease in the Minnesota business and professional men study, which started in 1947, he acknowledged that the Minnesota study was too small, and also did not follow a representative sample of men as most of the men were from a high socioeconomic level (discussed in chapter 1)[1]

Dr. Keys compared the Minnesota study with those of several other studies ongoing at the time, including the Framingham study. Dr. Keys entered all the data from his Minnesota subjects, data from the Framingham study (after 8 years of follow-up), and data from subjects from several other studies that were being conducted at the time, into a single table. When looking at the studies side by side, the conclusion was clear. In the last paragraph of the article, Dr. Keys wrote, "Comparison with similar follow-up data from Framingham, Massachusetts, Albany, New York, and Chicago, show a high degree of concordance. In all studies relative weight had least significance and the incidence of coronary heart disease rose continuously with the serum cholesterol level."[2]

Of course, Ancel Keys went on to set up the Seven Countries Study, but Dr. Keys's work prior to the Seven Countries Study was philosophically important in the design of the Framingham study, which was an epidemiological study to discover risk factors that contributed to the development of coronary heart disease.

Why Was the Framingham Study Conducted?

Just recently, as it approached its 65th anniversary, two histories of the Framingham Study were published.[3] [4]

1. Keys A, Blackburn HW, Taylor HL, Brožek J, Anderson JT, Simonson E. (1963) Coronary heart disease among Minnesota business and professional men followed fifteen years. *Circulation* 28: 381–395. http://www.ncbi.nlm.nih.gov/pubmed/?term=14059458
2. Ibid., page 393.
3. Oppenheimer GM. (2010) Framingham Heart Study: the first 20 years. *Prog Cardiovasc Dis* 53(1): 55-61. http://www.sciencedirect.com/science/article/pii/S0033062010000551

The Framingham Study had its roots in the heart disease suffered by President Franklin D. Roosevelt and the masses of Americans with heart disease (roughly half of all Americans) at that time. In 1948, President Harry Truman "signed into law, the National Heart Act," which was enacted because "the Nation's health is seriously threatened by diseases of the heart and circulation, including high blood pressure..."[5] The National Heart Institute chose the city of Framingham, Massachusetts, as the site of the study because it was a small city comprised mainly of middle-class residents of predominantly European origin (which resembled the population of the United States at the time), and it was also close to Boston and the expertise of the Harvard Medical School.

The plan was to recruit 6,000 out of the 10,000 adult residents of Framingham and follow them for as long as possible to determine what biological factors were important in the development of coronary heart disease. The first enrollees were examined on September 29, 1948.

By 1952 the first cohort of 5,209 residents had been recruited, and the first major scientific finding from the study was published in 1957.[6] The article reported that coronary heart disease was four times higher in residents with high blood pressure compared to residents with normal blood pressure, an observation that was quite unique at the time. Several hundred scientific papers have now been published from the Framingham Study.

In 1971 the Framingham Study commenced the recruitment of the children of the original residents and their spouses. In 1994 a survey study of the lipid and lipoprotein levels in the first generation offspring was published.[7]

4. Mahmood SS, Levy D, Vasan RS, Wang TJ. (2014) The Framingham Heart Study and the epidemiology of cardiovascular disease: a historical perspective. *Lancet* 383(9921): 999-1008. http://www.sciencedirect.com/science/article/pii/S0140673613617523#
5. Ibid., page 1000.
6. Ibid., page 1002.

The second and third directors of the Framingham study (Thomas Dawber, M.D., William Kannel, M.D.) were determined to find out how to prevent coronary heart disease, instead of finding treatments for patients who were already ill, as was the main emphasis in the practice of medicine at the time. In taking this approach, they were the first to use the term "risk factor" in their work and publications. The Framingham Risk Score later became the basis for the risk calculator used by the National Cholesterol Education Program.

The first major findings in the Framingham Study centered around the role of hypertension in the development of coronary heart disease. The investigators, who also studied how the heart itself changed with the disease, reported the novel finding that residents with asymptomatic left-ventricular systolic dysfunction suffered heart failure at greatly increased rates.

In addition to direct measures of heart health, the Framingham Study pioneered the use of metabolic risk factors to predict disease. Following the lead of Ancel Keys, the Framingham investigators measured serum cholesterol, and then, with ever increasing precision, went on to measure lipoprotein fractions. As early as 1952 the studies by Howard Eder's group showed that cholesterol in the alpha fraction was decreased in diseased states.[8] But these results were forgotten for some reason. In 1975 Miller and Miller published that high density lipoprotein (HDL) was involved in returning cholesterol to the liver and thus may be protective against coronary heart disease.[9] In 1977 investigators

7. Schaefer EJ, Lamon-Fava S, Cohn SD, Schaefer MM, Ordovas JM, Castelli WP, Wilson PWF. (1994) Effects of age, gender, and menopausal status on plasma low density lipoprotein cholesterol and apolipoprotein B levels in the Framingham Offspring Study. *J Lipid Res* 35: 779-792. http://www.jlr.org/content/35/5/779.long
8. Barr DP, Russ EM, Eder HA. (1951) Protein-lipid relationships in human plasma. II. In atherosclerosis and related conditions. *Am J Med 11*(4): 480-493.
9. Miller GJ, Miller NE. (1975) Plasma-high-density-lipoprotein concentration and development of ischaemic heart-disease. *Lancet* Jan 4;1(7897): 16-19.

from the Framingham Study reported the landmark observation that HDL cholesterol concentration was inversely related to the incidence of coronary heart disease.[10] This was a major advance in the study of lipid metabolism and the development of coronary heart disease.

The observations concerning HDL were not immediately reproduced, but eventually they were supported by other studies such as the results from the Lipid Research Clinics Coronary Primary Prevention Trial[11] and the PROCAM study performed in Germany.[12]

http://www.thelancet.com/journals/lancet/article/PIIS0140-6736%2875%2992376-4/abstract

10. Gordon T, Castelli WP, Hjortland MC, Kannel WB, Dawber TR. (1977) High density lipoprotein as a protective factor against coronary heart disease. The Framingham Study. *Am J Med* 62(5): 707-714. http://www.ncbi.nlm.nih.gov/pubmed/193398
11. Gordon DJ, Knoke J, Probstfield JL, Superko R, Tyroler HA. (1986) High-density lipoprotein cholesterol and coronary heart disease in hypercholesterolemic men: the Lipid Research Clinics Coronary Primary Prevention Trial. *Circulation* 74: 1217-1225.
12. Assmann G, Schulte H, von Eckardstein A, Huang Y. (1996) High-density lipoprotein cholesterol as a predictor of coronary heart disease risk. The PROCAM experience and pathophysiological implications for reverse cholesterol transport. *Atherosclerosis* 124 Suppl. S11-S20

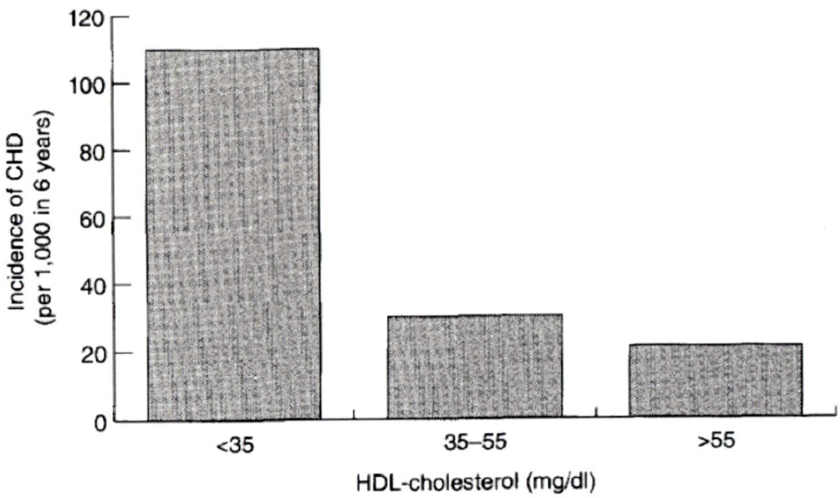

These data from the PROCAM study in Germany showed that a low HDL-cholesterol concentration was a strong risk factor for coronary heart disease. Figure from Assmann et al. (1996) Atherosclerosis 124: Suppl. S11-S20.

In 2015 we understand better the different functions of HDL and LDL in the movement of cholesterol throughout the body. Our current understanding of the known functions of these lipoproteins support the original observations from the Framingham Study.

In 2002 the Framingham Study began to recruit the third generation of participants, who are the grandchildren of the original residents. The multigenerational nature of the study lends itself to studies of the genetics of lipid metabolism and the development of coronary heart disease. Besides precisely defining the risk factor profiles for coronary heart disease, other major discoveries of the Framingham Study, as discussed in full by Mahmood *et al.*,[13] were:

13. Mahmood SS *et al.* See previous citation in this chapter.

1. 1971–Systolic pressure was superior to diastolic pressure in predicting coronary heart disease.[14]

2. 1974–Type 2 Diabetes mellitus increases coronary heart disease mortality [15]

See Mahmood *et al.*[16] to read about these other milestones:

3. 1978–Non-rheumatic atrial fibrillation is a risk factor for stroke.

4. 1985–Postmenopausal estrogen use and smoking are linked to coronary heart disease.

The observation from the Framingham Study that HDL was protective against coronary heart disease explained some of the anomalies in the cholesterol story that were widely debated in the nutrition and medical fields at the time. When serum cholesterol was very, very high, most likely the cause was an increase in LDL cholesterol. This corresponded with Ancel Keys's observations that very high cholesterol concentrations (> 220 mg/dL) were strongly correlated with coronary heart disease across many countries after only 10 years of follow-up.[17] With intermediate increases in cholesterol concentrations, the cholesterol in the blood could be the result of either increases in LDL cholesterol or HDL cholesterol, or both. Therefore, with the insertion of this extra complexity–that some cholesterol (LDL) is hazardous and other cholesterol (HDL) is protective–there was more variance in populations concerning the association of total cholesterol with coronary heart disease.

14. Kannel WB, Gordon T, Schwartz MJ. (1971) Systolic versus diastolic blood pressure and risk of coronary heart disease. The Framingham study. *Am J Cardiol* 27: 335–346. www.sciencedirect.com/science/article/pii/0002914971904280
15. Garcia MJ, McNamara PM, Gordon T, Kannel WB. (1974) Morbidity and mortality in diabetics in the Framingham population. Sixteen year follow-up study. *Diabetes* 23: 105–111. http://diabetes.diabetesjournals.org/content/23/2/105.long
16. Mahmood SS *et al.* See previous citation in this chapter.
17. Keys A. *et al.* (1980) Seven Countries. A multivariate analysis of death and coronary heart disease. Cambridge, MA: Harvard University Press. (See full citation in chapter 1)

In fact, in some of the later reports from the Framingham Study,[18] when the total cholesterol value was divided by the HDL cholesterol, the resulting value was a much better predictor of coronary heart disease than using LDL cholesterol only.

This was confirmed recently[19] by a study that was designed to test which lipoprotein or cholesterol parameter was more precise in its predictive value of coronary heart disease. Total cholesterol/ HDL cholesterol was still as good as any other clinical chemistry measurement that is currently being performed in predicting the probability of coronary heart disease.

What is HDL?

HDL is a lipoprotein totally distinct from LDL and contains a different structural protein, apolipoprotein A-I (apoA-I), which is secreted relatively lipid poor[20] from both liver and the intestine and picks up lipid as it circulates in blood. The structure of HDL has been studied for over 20 years and several models of the lipoprotein have been produced. The model of HDL that I use throughout this book is the one devised in the laboratory of Dr. Klaus Schulten.[21] In the following figure a discoidal HDL is shown with two apoA-I proteins that surround the particle in a planar, belt-like orientation. The phospholipid molecules (approximately 160 in number) form the top and bottom caps with their fatty

18. Schaefer EJ et al. (1994) (See full citation earlier in chapter).
19. Ingelsson E, Schaefer EJ, Contois JH, McNamara JR, Sullivan L, Keyes MJ, Pencina MJ, Schoonmaker C, Wilson PW, D'Agostino RB, Vasan RS. (2007) Clinical utility of different lipid measures for prediction of coronary heart disease in men and women. *JAMA* 298(7): 776-785. http://jama.jamanetwork.com/article.aspx?articleid=208432
20. Dixon JL, Battini R, Ferrari S, Redman CM, Banerjee D. (1989) Expression and secretion of chicken apolipoprotein AI in transfected COS cells. *Biochim Biophys Acta* 1009(1): 47-53. http://www.sciencedirect.com/science/article/pii/0167478189900778
21. Diagram of HDL courtesy of Dr. Klaus Schulten, Beckman Institute for Advanced Science and Technology, and Department of Physics, University of Illinois at Urbana-Champaign, Urbana, IL 61801, USA. http://www.ks.uiuc.edu/Research/Lipoproteins/

acyl chains (in orange-gold) directed down and up into the core of the molecule. This discoidal HDL carries only a small number of cholesterol molecules. Such discoidal HDL particles have been observed in electron micrographs of concentrated HDL.

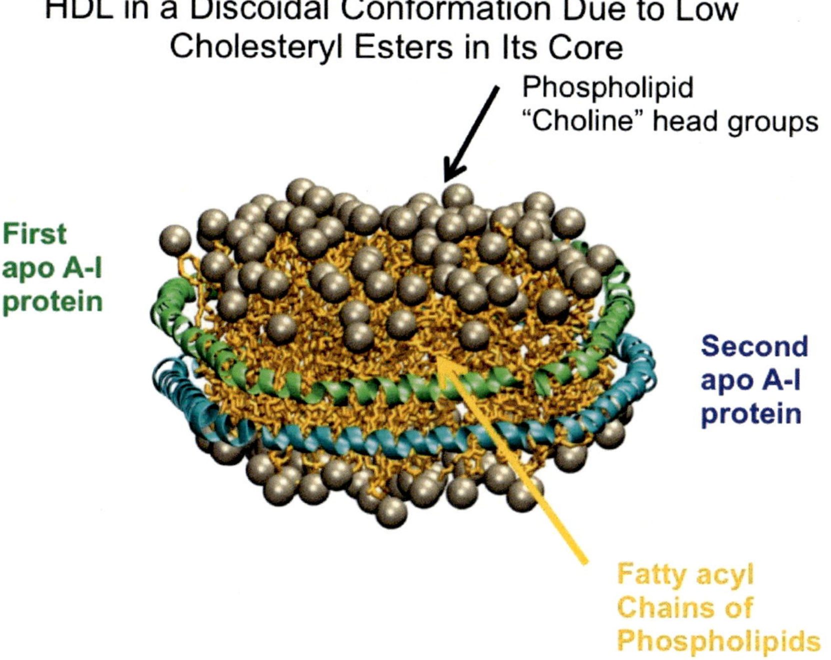

Diagram of HDL in the discoid conformation containing only small amounts of cholesteryl ester. Two copies of the protein, apolipoprotein A-I, wrap around the particle in a belt-like configuration. Courtesy of Dr. Klaus Schulten of the Beckman Institute for Advanced Science and Technology, and Department of Physics, University of Illinois at Urbana-Champaign, Urbana. http://www.ks.uiuc.edu/Research/Lipoproteins/

In the next figure the HDL particle (now depicted as a grey background) is modeled picking up cholesteryl ester molecules (starting with 6 and ending with 60 molecules), and as it obtains more and more cholesteryl esters, the shape of the particle changes from a disc to a spherical particle.[22] In this figure the elongated color molecules (representing individual cholesteryl esters) diffuse into the particle and form the core of the HDL spherical particle. In this way HDL can pick up excess cholesterol from peripheral tissues and carry them back to the liver in a process termed reverse cholesterol transport.

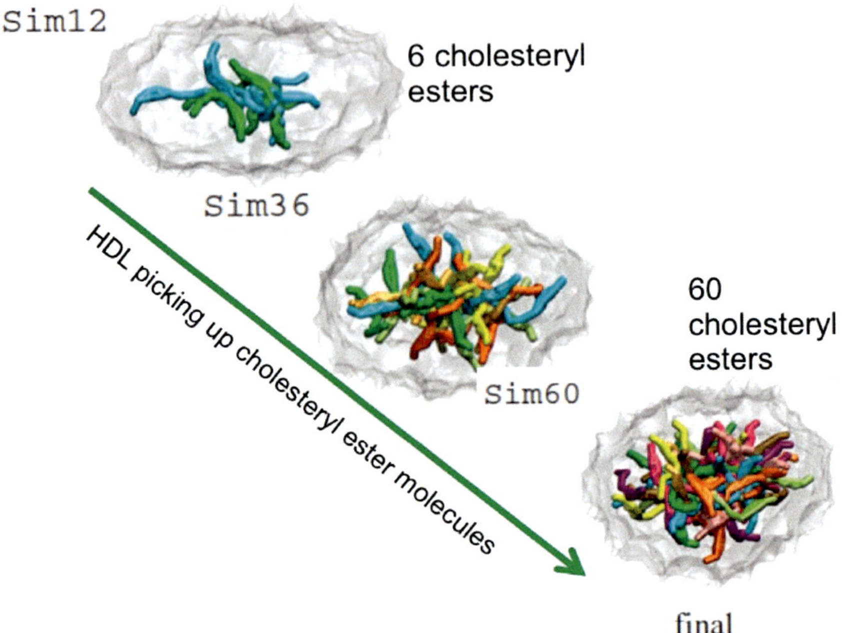

A HDL disc particle (now depicted as a grey background) is modeled picking up cholesteryl ester molecules, and as it obtains more and more molecules, the shape of the particle changes from a disc to a spherical particle. The elongated color molecules represent individual cholesteryl esters, which diffuse into the particle to form the core of the HDL spherical particle. Courtesy of Dr. Klaus Schulten of the Beckman Institute for Advanced Science and Technology, and Department of Physics, University of Illinois at Urbana-Champaign, Urbana. http://www.ks.uiuc.edu/Research/Lipoproteins/

22. Shih AY, Sligar SG, Schulten, K. (2009) Maturation of high-density lipoproteins. *J Royal Soc Interface* 6, 863–871. http://www.ncbi.nlm.nih.gov/pmc/articles/PMC2805102/

A full review article on the structure of HDL has been published that presents multiple lines of evidence for the model of HDL that contains the apoA-I proteins in an "anti-parallel, double-belt conformation around the edge of the disc" of the HDL particle. [23]

What Was Learned about Blood Lipids and Lipoproteins from the Framingham Study and Subsequent Studies?

We now know that there are two major pools of cholesterol in blood, with high levels of cholesterol in LDL being hazardous and high levels of cholesterol in HDL being protective.

23. Phillips MC (2013) New insights into the determination of HDL structure by apolipoproteins: Thematic review series: high density lipoprotein structure, function, and metabolism. *J Lipid Res* 54(8): 2034-2048. http://www.jlr.org/content/54/8/2034.long

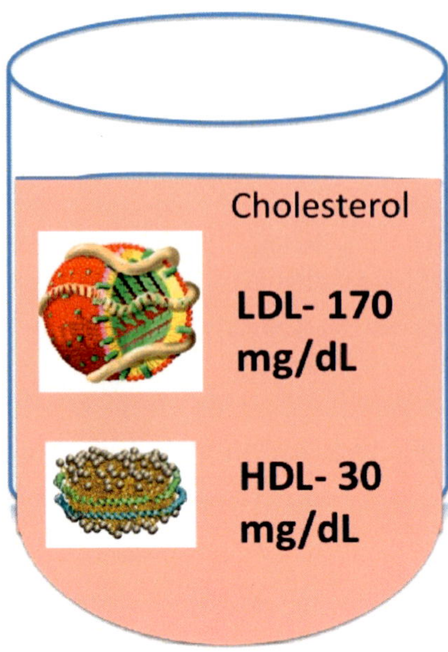

A person with a high total cholesterol (240 mg/dL) may have the following distribution between LDL and HDL in blood;
Total C/HDL C = 8
High Risk Factor for CHD

Depiction of the two lipoproteins (LDL and HDL) in blood. In the example LDL carries 73% of the total blood cholesterol and HDL carries only 13%. The remaining cholesterol is distributed among other lipoproteins or their remnants.

Additional studies defined the roles of LDL and HDL lipoproteins. Below is a concise summary of their metabolism and roles.

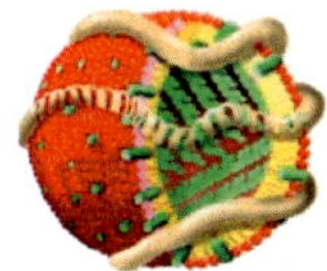
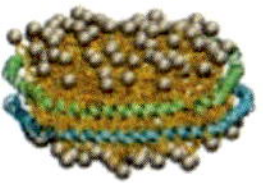

Name	LDL	HDL
Carries	Cholesterol (esters)	Cholesterol (esters)
Main Protein	ApoB	ApoA-I
Diameter (in nanometers)	24	10
Function in Body	Carries cholesterol to many tissues	Brings cholesterol back to liver
Derived from	VLDL	ApoA-I Secreted by liver and intestine; cholesterol is from peripheral tissues
High Levels	Risk Factor for CHD	Protective against CHD
Nick name	Bad Cholesterol	Good Cholesterol

Comparison of the characteristics and functions of LDL and HDL.

Roles of LDL and HDL in the Blood

Most LDL is formed from very low density lipoprotein (VLDL), which is secreted by the liver. If LDL in blood is very high, LDL is able to enter the artery wall of the major conduit arteries of the heart. HDL, which is mostly formed in blood after initial secretion of its main structural protein ApoA-I by liver or intestine, permeates throughout the blood of the body and scours up any extra cholesterol molecules (like a cholesterol vacuum cleaner) and delivers them back to the liver.[24] For many decades HDL keeps the levels of cholesterol in the arteries low enough to prevent their progression to full blown coronary heart disease. As with LDL receptors, the HDL concentration declines with age, thereby allowing atherosclerotic disease to progress in older

24. Rosenson RS, Brewer HB Jr, Davidson WS, Fayad ZA, Fuster V, Goldstein J, Hellerstein M, Jiang XC, Phillips MC, Rader DJ, Remaley AT, Rothblat GH, Tall AR, Yvan-Charvet L. (2012) Cholesterol efflux and atheroprotection: advancing the concept of reverse cholesterol transport. *Circulation* 125(15): 1905-1919. http://circ.ahajournals.org/content/125/15/1905.long

humans. Of course, humans with a low HDL from birth have a higher risk for coronary heart disease than humans who have a high HDL throughout their lives.

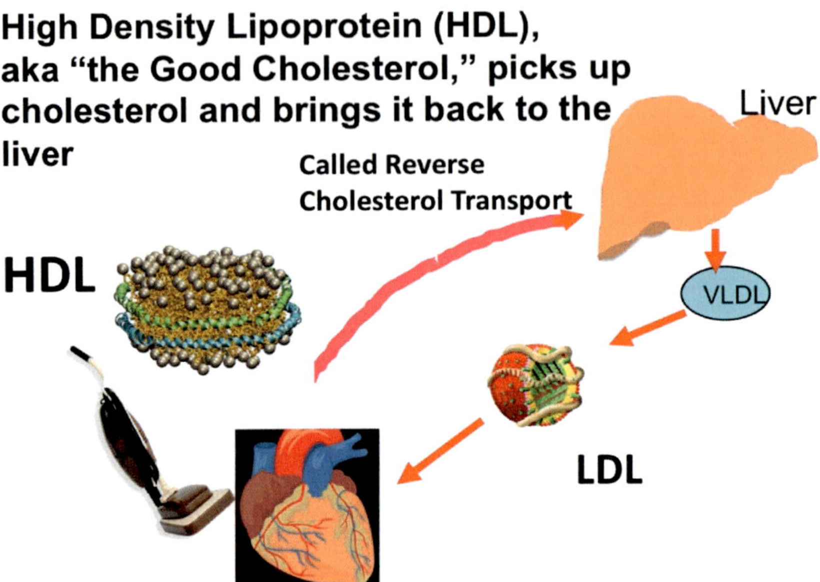

HDL, which has apolipoprotein AI as a structural protein, is completely different from the apolipoprotein B family of lipoproteins, which includes VLDL and LDL. HDL, secreted lipid-poor from the liver and small intestine, permeates through the blood stream and picks up excess cholesterol from tissues, including the coronary arteries of the heart, and delivers it back to the liver. Because of this function, the actions of HDL resemble that of a vacuum cleaner for cholesterol.

Below is a theoretical breakdown of LDL and HDL cholesterol concentrations in blood from two individuals with either a low or high total cholesterol concentration. The blood with low total cholesterol concentration contains optimal levels of LDL and HDL cholesterol, compared to the high serum total cholesterol, which contains levels of LDL and HDL cholesterol that would indicate a high risk for coronary heart disease. At the bottom, the total cholesterol/HDL cholesterol is calculated and the person with a high cholesterol example presents with an extremely high ratio value of 8.

Theoretical Blood Lipoproteins at Different Total Cholesterol Levels:

	Total cholesterol (mg/dL) Low	High
Total cholesterol	140	240
LDL cholesterol (Atherogenic) 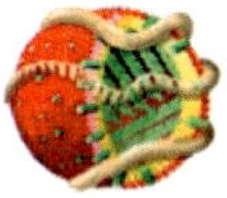	80	170
HDL cholestero (Protective) 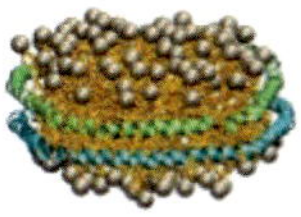	50	30
Total cholesterol (TC) / HDL cholesterol	2.8	8

TC/HDL-C >5 is a powerful risk factor

Theoretical blood lipoprotein cholesterol distributions. The person on the left with the low total cholesterol concentration (140 mg/dL) has a low LDL cholesterol (80 mg/dL) and a reasonably high HDL cholesterol (50 mg/dL) concentration. The person on the right with a high total cholesterol concentration has a high LDL cholesterol (170 mg/dL) and a low HDL cholesterol (30 mg/dL). The person with the cholesterol distribution on the right would be considered to have a higher risk for coronary heart disease.

As the 1980s were approaching, more and more information was becoming available concerning risk factors for coronary heart disease. The Seven Countries Study was responsible for showing that diet had a significant influence on coronary heart disease. The Framingham Study more precisely defined the lipoprotein profiles that were either protective or hazardous.

However, there were still many other factors that could influence health and disease. Exercise was protective but it needed to be performed throughout life. And as discussed in the previous chapters, other constituents in the diet such as fiber have effects (most likely indirectly) on the development of coronary heart disease.[25] But in the 1980s, most of the metabolic experimental evidence that was known concerned lipids. Many other discoveries were yet to come.

25. http://www.health.gov/dietaryguidelines/dga2005/report/HTML/table_d5_1.htm

13.

DISCOVERY OF THE STATIN DRUGS, ROLLBACK OF LDL, AND PROTECTION FROM CHD

What Are the Causes of Coronary Heart Disease (CHD)?

The prevailing hypothesis right now is that coronary heart disease is caused by high levels of LDL over many years, although, as will be discussed in the next chapter, other biological factors can either enhance the damage LDL causes or protect against excess LDL, or even, cause coronary heart disease directly.

As I described earlier, LDL is a lipid droplet surrounded by a structural protein. The lipid droplet mainly carries cholesterol in the form of esters, and there are about 1,500 cholesteryl ester molecules per LDL particle.

The most agreed upon mechanism (and this is still being debated by scientists) how an increased blood LDL concentration causes coronary arteries to become blocked is that LDL invades the area under the endothelial cell lining of the arteries (see following figure).[1] [2] This area, called the subendothelial space, becomes infiltrated with LDL particles, and immune cells (monocytes/macrophages), which are charged with keeping the subendothelial space clean. In most of us, for much of the first 30-40 years of life, HDL particles efficiently return excess cholesterol to the liver for disposal and the plaque remains small and benign. But over decades, after the blood LDL cholesterol starts to increase, the process of cleaning out the subendothelial space can be overwhelmed, and cholesterol, debris, foam cells (engorged macrophages), and other constituents can accumulate in the artery wall and partially block the lumen (opening) of the artery.

1. Wong BW, Meredith A, Lin D, McManus BM (2012) The Biological Role of Inflammation in Atherosclerosis. *Canadian Journal of Cardiology*, 28(6): 631–641. http://www.sciencedirect.com/science/article/pii/S0828282X12003261
2. Rosenfeld ME. (2013) Inflammation and atherosclerosis: direct versus indirect mechanisms. *Curr Opin Pharmacol* 13(2): 154-160. http://www.sciencedirect.com/science/article/pii/S1471489213000076

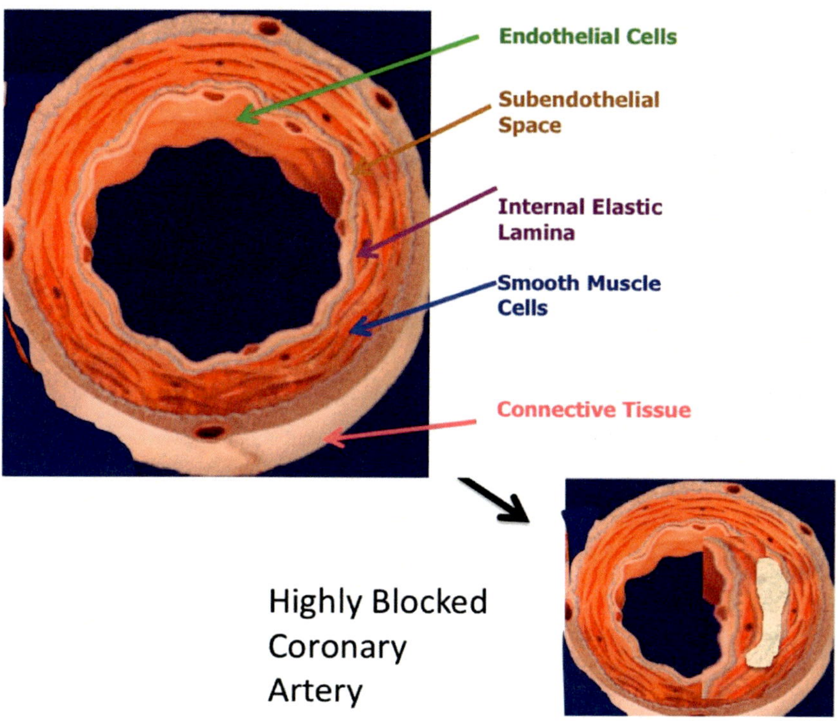

Overtime, a clean coronary artery can become blocked due to the development of an atherosclerotic plaque. The precise mechanism how this occurs is still being investigated as it is difficult to study a process that may take 20 to 30 years to occur in a human artery.

A heart attack occurs when the artery is mostly or totally occluded. This occurs most often when a plaque from another region of the circulation ruptures and travels to the site of the partial blockage and causes a total or near total blockage of the coronary artery. When blood cannot flow to certain areas of the heart, heart muscle cells in that region do not receive enough oxygen and die. This basic mechanism is extremely complex and involves many different cell types and a multitude of proteins and signaling molecules. To this day, the precise steps have not been worked out and active research is being conducted on this mechanism by many different laboratories.

The experimental evidence that LDL causes coronary heart disease was developed over a 50-60-year period after the discovery of the lipoprotein families and the development of methods used to isolate lipoproteins and study them and their metabolism.

Brown and Goldstein's work[3] with patients with familial hypercholesterolemia, some of whom died of heart attacks as early as six years old, showed that defects in the LDL receptor of cells were often responsible for the very high buildup of LDL in blood in these patients.

What about the rest of us–those without a genetic hyperlipidemia? As also discussed earlier, the LDL receptor number or activity decreases with age. When combined with an atherogenic diet or with some other risk factor, the likelihood of developing coronary heart disease increases as we become older.

The Discovery of Statins

What to do about cholesterol and increased coronary heart disease in the rest of us was answered with a scientific discovery made by Akira Endo in Japan.[4] Dr. Endo worked for Sankyo Chemical Company and he was interested in finding an inhibitor of cholesterol synthesis in fungi, just as penicillin had been discovered and isolated from the fungus, *Penicillium notatum*. After testing many different preparations from different fungi, Dr. Endo finally isolated a compound from *Penicillium citrinum* that could inhibit the enzyme hydroxy methylglutaryl-Coenzyme A reductase, a key enzyme in the cholesterol synthesis pathway. Once the structure of the compound was determined, it was called

3. Goldstein JL, Brown MS. (2009) The LDL receptor. *Arterioscler Thromb Vasc Biol* 29(4): 431-438. http://atvb.ahajournals.org/content/29/4/431.long
4. Li, Jie Jack (2009) Triumph of the Heart: The Story of Statins. Oxford University Press.

mevastatin (also called compactin) due to its similarity to mevalonate, an intermediate in the cholesterol synthesis pathway. Sankyo Chemical Company then enticed Merck and Company in the United States to become interested in mevastatin and take over the research and development.

Using data and insights into mevastatin from Sankyo, scientists at Merck isolated from a different fungus a very similar compound that was a slightly more powerful inhibitor of cholesterol synthesis than mevastatin. This second compound was call lovastatin and, after clinical studies, it was approved by the Food and Drug Administration in 1987 for the treatment of hypercholesterolemia, and became the first prescription statin drug, known as Mevacor, to be available in the United States.

What Dr. Endo had discovered in the fungus was an active ingredient (mevastatin or compactin) that was capable of binding to and stopping the enzyme, hydroxy methylglutaryl-Coenzyme A reductase, one of the early enzymes in the complicated pathway of cholesterol synthesis. The following figure gives clues to how mevastatin works. Mevastatin was extracted from the fungus and a portion of the molecule remarkably resembles the configuration of mevalonate, an intermediate in cholesterol synthesis. When the drug mevastatin enters a cell, it binds to hydroxy methylglutaryl-Coenzyme A reductase, which carries out the reaction that produces mevalonate from the enzyme's substrate, hydroxymethyl glutaryl Coenzyme A. Mevastatin prevents mevalonate from being formed in the reaction from the natural substrate, and this inhibits cholesterol synthesis. As you might expect, the tighter an inhibitor like mevastatin can bind to the enzyme, the more effective the inhibitor will be.

When studies noted that mevastatin could decrease LDL in the blood of humans, many pharmaceutical companies developed research programs to find compounds that were similar to but more powerful than mevastatin. Therefore, as shown in the following figure, pharmaceutical companies developed a series of compounds that were very similar to mevastatin (compactin), but that bound tighter to the hydroxy methylglutaryl-Coenzyme A reductase enzyme targeted in the pathway.

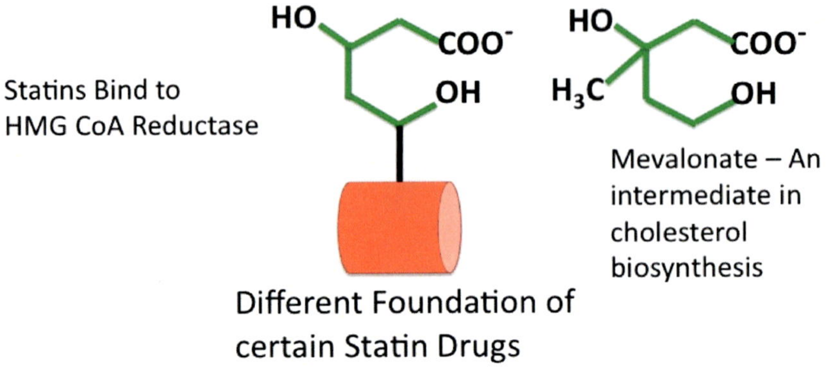

Statins Bind to
HMG CoA Reductase

HO
COO^-
OH

HO
COO^-
H_3C
OH

Mevalonate – An intermediate in cholesterol biosynthesis

Different Foundation of certain Statin Drugs

Statin drugs are inhibitors of cholesterol synthesis and the following have a portion of their structures that resemble mevalonate, an intermediate in the cholesterol biosynthetic pathway: compactin, lovastatin (Mevacor), pravastatin (Pravachol), and simvastatin (Zocor).

Thus, once the original chemical was isolated from the fungus and shown to be effective, pharmaceutical company chemists worked to alter the structure slightly in order to improve the drug. This explains the rapid development of an array of more potent statin drugs during the 20-year period after mevastatin was discovered in Dr. Endo's fungal preparation. Several companies were indeed very successful and now this class of pharmaceuticals, known collectively as statins, is one of the most prescribed drugs in the entire world.

But How Do Statins Lower Blood LDL?

The mechanism by which statin drugs lower LDL cholesterol, and thus total cholesterol in blood, is an interesting one. Although hydroxy methylglutaryl-Coenzyme A reductase is present in almost all cells, it is the enzyme in liver cells that is especially important for the regulation of blood LDL concentrations. As demonstrated in the following figure, after the statin binds to hydroxy methylglutaryl-Coenzyme A reductase in liver cells, it inhibits the synthesis of cholesterol (represented by the large cross bars in liver) in the liver. Lower cholesterol levels within liver cells (shown as a whole liver in the figure) are sensed, and the cells increase the synthesis of LDL receptors, which go to the cell membrane. The increased number of LDL receptors take up more LDL from blood so that the liver cells can have enough cholesterol for their membranes and other pathways. In a sense, statins "trick" the liver into taking up more LDL from the blood, preventing higher LDL concentrations in blood and excess LDL from invading the arteries of the heart.

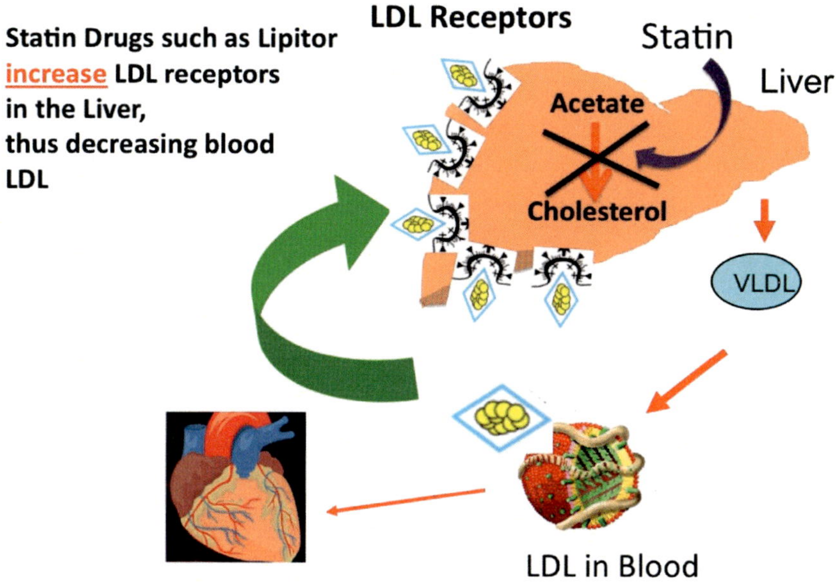

Statin drugs inhibit cholesterol synthesis in liver and this results in increased numbers of LDL receptors on the surface of liver cells. The increased LDL receptors take up more LDL from blood, thus lowering LDL cholesterol in blood.

What Have the Clinical Trials Told Us about Statins?

In 2010, a meta analysis[5] of 21 trials involving statins versus placebo (129,526 individuals; median follow-up 4.8 years) and five additional studies that tested an aggressive statin dose versus a lower statin dose, indicated that statin therapy caused an all-cause mortality decrease of 10% per 1.0 mmol/L (equivalent to a decrease in 39 mg of cholesterol) drop in blood LDL concentration. The decrease in mortality was largely due to decreased coronary heart disease. Therefore, for every decrease in 1 mmol/L (39 mg/dL) of LDL cholesterol, a 10% reduction in coronary heart disease is expected. The large number of subjects in these clinical trials put to rest the nagging questions of whether statins increased deaths due to cancer or other nonvascular causes. The answer was that they did not. Statins are fairly safe drugs, although side effects such as muscle pain are certainly a possibility.

Why do some people not show increased blood cholesterol with an atherogenic diet or with increasing age?

The observation that some individuals are not sensitive to diets high in saturated fat and dietary cholesterol that increase serum cholesterol in most people have now been explained by the discovery of PCSK9, a protein that is involved in diverting LDL receptors for degradation inside cells (especially liver cells).[6] When the PCSK9 protein is mutated, individuals have more LDL receptors than usual on the membranes of their liver cells. Approximately one out of 30 persons have one allele (for most

5. Cholesterol Treatment Trialists' (CTT) Collaboration. (2010) Efficacy and safety of more intensive lowering of LDL cholesterol: a meta-analysis of data from 170, 000 participants in 26 randomised trials. *Lancet* 376: 1670–1681.
6. Seidah NG, Awan Z, Chrétien M, Mbikay M. (2014) PCSK9: a key modulator of cardiovascular health. *Circ Res* 114(6): 1022-1036.

genes, each person has a copy of the gene (an allele) from each parent) coding for a mutation in the PCSK9 protein, such that blood LDL cholesterol concentration is decreased by about 15% and coronary heart disease is lowered by about 45% in these people. Individuals with both PCSK9 alleles mutated have much higher numbers of LDL receptors on their cell membranes and, therefore, much lower LDL cholesterol concentrations (decreased by 40%). These lucky individuals present with a 90% decrease in coronary heart disease. The presiding interpretation is that lifelong loss of PCSK9 protein leads to low blood LDL over a lifetime, and this causes very strong protection against LDL-directed plaque development, and results in much lower rates of coronary heart disease. A small percentage of unlucky individuals have higher PCSK9 activity, and thus, they have higher LDL cholesterol levels and increased risk for coronary heart disease.

The PCSK9 story illustrates that the basic mechanism for removing LDL from the blood using the LDL receptor, as originally determined by Goldstein and Brown, was correct, but that genetic diversity led to more complicated regulation than originally conceived by early researchers. The PCSK9 story also reinforces the central role of LDL cholesterol levels in the basic etiology of coronary heart disease.

Many studies by investigators all over the world have given support to Ancel Keys's original observation–that blood cholesterol levels, especially very high blood cholesterol concentrations, are associated with coronary heart disease. In fact, as shown in later studies, LDL cholesterol was shown to be a direct player in increasing the development of coronary artery plaques. There is certainly evidence, that will be discussed in the next chapter, that other factors play a role in the development of coronary heart disease, such that some people with low LDL concentrations may develop disease. The differences in biological variability among humans, even within fairly well defined and stable populations, are quite wide, such that making a precise, accurate prediction concerning whether a specific individual will develop coronary heart disease is extremely difficult.

14.

EVEN WHEN YOUR CHOLESTEROL LEVELS ARE PERFECT, AVOID THAT SECOND SLICE OF CHEESECAKE

One day I was taking a break from swimming in the pool when the fellow in the next lane struck up a conversation. He told me how he had a heart attack eight months earlier. He was now swimming to stay in shape. Before his heart attack his doctor had told him that his lipids were perfect! Therefore, he did not watch what he ate and he would always go for that second slice of cheesecake! Now everything was different. Besides exercise, he was now on a strict diet and watched everything he ate. Then he turned to me and said, “But my doctor said my lipids were perfect and I still had a heart attack. Can you believe it?”

Actually, I can. If you understand lipid metabolism you can imagine how such a thing is possible.

The swimmer’s story illustrates some of the criticisms of the lipid hypothesis concerning coronary heart disease. The Framingham Study showed us that the blood LDL cholesterol concentration was just the tip of one iceberg among many risk factor icebergs. And the process of coronary heart disease development is extremely complex and occurs slowly over many years. In fact, there are several biological avenues, distinct from LDL, that can lead to increased atherosclerosis in the main coronary conduit arteries.

The experience of the Finns in East Finland, after the realization that their diet was leading to increased coronary heart disease, is probably the strongest data we have indicating that a high-saturated fat-diet, along with a diet low in plant materials, leads to high blood cholesterol levels and high coronary heart disease.[1] When the Finns changed their diet, treated high blood pressure, and decreased smoking, their coronary heart disease rates decreased to 50% of the rates originally observed by Ancel Keys and Martti Karvonen in the late 1950-early 1960s.

But the coronary heart disease rate still remained relatively above control for some years as it is difficult to reverse atherosclerosis after someone has been eating a poor diet for many years. With the newer generation statin drugs, it is possible to cause regression of plaques with aggressive therapy that decreases LDL to very low levels (LDL cholesterol of approximately 70 mg/dL or lower). However, therapy for high blood lipids is beyond the scope of this book.

It is also the case that many other biological processes, besides high LDL cholesterol, are involved in the development of atherosclerosis. Let's review some of the biological mechanisms that are now being investigated for their effects on the development of plaques in the coronary arteries. The following

1. Oppenheimer GM, Blackburn H, Puska, P. (2011) From Framingham to North Karelia to U.S. Community-Based prevention programs: negotiating research agenda for coronary heart disease in the second half of the 20th Century. *Public Health Reviews* 33(2): 450-483. http://www.publichealthreviews.eu/show/i/10

figure shows that there are many biological factors that affect the health of the artery. On the left is a spanking clean artery, and on the right is an artery that has an atherosclerotic plaque. The surrounding arrows on the left show the biological processes that influence and stimulate plaque development. LDL-cholesterol is just one factor. Other factors are listed below.

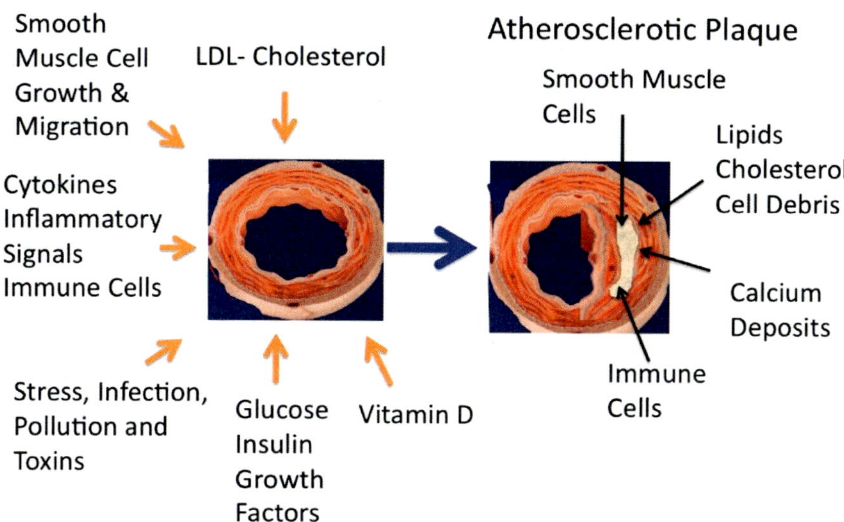

Many different biological processes can contribute to the development of an atherosclerotic plaque. On the left is a vessel without plaque; on the right is a vessel that has a mature plaque made up of deposited lipids, smooth muscle cells that have moved into the subendothelial space, immune cells, and calcium deposits.

Diabetes and Other Pro-atherogenic Factors

Diabetes also has a very strong effect on coronary arteries. In fact, at each level of cholesterol concentration in the blood, diabetics have four times the rate of coronary heart disease compared to nondiabetics.[2] This indicates that diabetes provides a very strong additional damaging effect on the artery above that provided by LDL cholesterol. How diabetes increases heart attacks is a major research area in medicine. As described below, diabetes influences the cells of the coronary artery in a sinister way.

Smooth Muscle Cell Growth and Migration

Smooth muscle cells surround the endothelial cells, the subendothelial space, and the internal elastic lamina that line the artery lumen (See first image in Chapter 13). Just like regular muscle, smooth muscle cells can either contract or dilate in order to change the area of the opening. For reasons that we do not understand, smooth muscle cells can turn proliferative and begin to divide.[3] Then with the help of an enzyme called MMP-9, a protease that can chew through matrix, smooth muscle cells begin to migrate and can move into the subendothelial space or even into the lumen of the artery.

The image below shows a coronary artery from a diabetic pig that had been fed a diet containing a high-saturated-fat, high-cholesterol content.[4] The lumen of the artery is almost completely occluded because smooth muscle cells, immune cells, and lipids have expanded the subendothelial space. In fact, the coronary artery lesions observed in pig hearts are very similar to the lesions that develop in human coronary arteries. This is one

2. Chait A, Bornfeldt KE. (2009) Diabetes and atherosclerosis: is there a role for hyperglycemia? *J Lipid Res* 50 Suppl:S335-S339. http://www.jlr.org/content/50/Supplement/S335.long
3. Johnson JL. (2014) Emerging regulators of vascular smooth muscle cell function in the development and progression of atherosclerosis. *Cardiovasc Res 103*(4): 452-460. http://cardiovascres.oxfordjournals.org/content/103/4/452.long
4. Dixon JL, Shen S, Vuchetich JP, Wysocka E, Sun GY, Sturek M. (2002) Increased atherosclerosis in diabetic dyslipidemic swine: protection by atorvastatin involves decreased VLDL triglycerides but minimal effects on the lipoprotein profile. *J Lipid Res* 43(10): 1618-1629. http://www.jlr.org/content/43/10/1618.long

of the reasons why we employed pigs in our studies of coronary heart disease development in diabetes. What is extremely interesting about this lesion in the artery is that it is largely cellular and not overwhelmed with "foam cells" or lipid deposits.

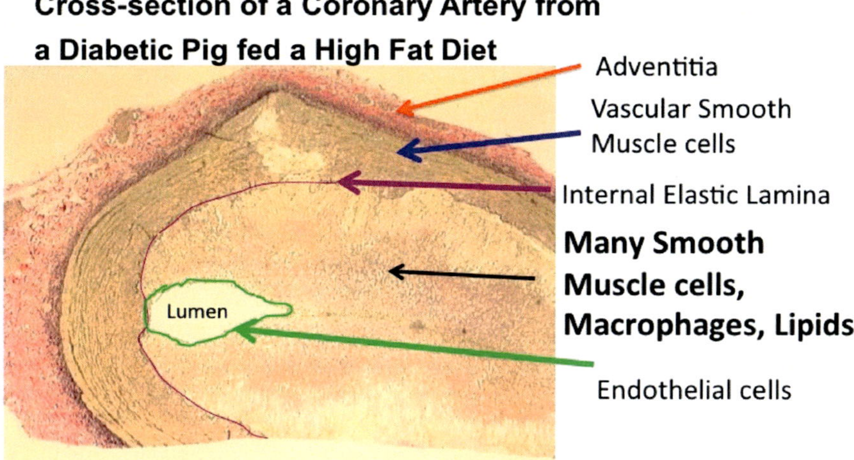

Section of a coronary artery from a diabetic pig fed a high saturated fat, high cholesterol diet. The section was stained using Verhoff-van Giesen elastin stain. The subendothelial space in the artery wall was filled with infiltrating smooth muscle cells, macrophages, and lipid (determined with specific stains). Courtesy of Michael Sturek and JL Dixon.

The laboratory of Michael Sturek has been exploring the health of coronary artery vascular smooth muscle cells for over 20 years in order to determine what causes these cells to divide and migrate in atherosclerosis. Dr. Sturek's studies have established that calcium metabolism is highly dysregulated in vascular smooth muscle cells in coronary artery disease.[5] Changes in calcium signaling alters gene expression leading to the proliferation and

5. Sturek M. (2011) Ca2+ regulatory mechanisms of exercise protection against coronary artery disease in metabolic syndrome and diabetes. *J Applied Physiol* 111: 573–586. http://jap.physiology.org/content/111/2/573

migration of smooth muscle cells throughout the artery. As observed in the cross section of the coronary artery in the above figure, the movement of smooth muscle cells contributes to the development of coronary artery plaques. In particular, Dr. Sturek has documented multiple changes in calcium metabolism in vascular muscle cells in diabetes, including impaired Ca2+ extrusion via the cell membrane Ca2+ ATPase, downregulated L-type voltage-gated Ca2+ channels, increased Ca2+ sequestration by the sarcoplasmic reticulum Ca2+ ATPase (known as SERCA), and increased accumulation of Ca2+ within the cell nucleus.

Immune System and Inflammatory Response

Another factor involved in plaque development is the immune system and its powerful taskmaster, the inflammatory response, which is now considered a central mediator of atherosclerosis. As stated by one group of researchers, "Inflammation initiates, propagates, and complicates the course of atherosclerosis. A multitude of basic science work demonstrates this pathophysiological principle."[6]

An important aspect of the inflammatory response is the recruitment of immune cells to the location where the atherosclerotic plaque is growing. The reason for this is that the body wishes to repair the artery. But what really happens is that the immune cells will overreact and damage the artery. The inflammatory response is thought to be behind the damaging effects of stress, infection, pollution, and toxins.

Vitamin D

There have been reports that low levels of vitamin D metabolites are associated with increased rates of coronary heart disease.[7]

6. Wolf D, Stachon P, Bode C, Zirlik A. (2014) Inflammatory mechanisms in atherosclerosis *Hämostaseologie* 1: 63-71. http://www.schattauer.de/en/magazine/subject-areas/journals-a-z/haemostaseologie/contents/archive/issue/1830.html

In a prospective epidemiological study of 3,258 patients, mean age of 62 years and followed for a mean of 7.7 years, low concentrations of 25-hydroxyvitamin D and 1,25-dihydroxyvitamin D, active metabolites of vitamin D, were associated with higher rates of all-cause and cardiovascular death in both men and women. This study, carried out in Germany, was the first prospective cohort study that showed a strong protective effect of vitamin D metabolites against cardiovascular disease.[8] Low vitamin D action may cause cells in the artery to lay down calcium phosphate, thus leading to the calcium buildup observed in advanced plaque regions. Additionally, low vitamin D availability may be involved in increased inflammation.[9] The detrimental effects of low vitamin D metabolites on cardiovascular disease may be the result of high blood parathyroid hormone concentrations, a condition that occurs when vitamin D is low.[10] [11] Therefore, the extra levels of sunshine that people in the Mediterranean area receive the year round may increase vitamin D production in the skin. This would lead to greater activity of vitamin D-dependent processes and thus contribute to artery health, and possibly influence rates of coronary heart disease. This is another reason why the intake

7. Kassi E, Adamopoulos C, Basdra EK, Papavassiliou AG. (2013) Role of vitamin D in atherosclerosis. *Circulation* 128(23): 2517-2531. http://www.ncbi.nlm.nih.gov/pubmed/24297817
8. Dobnig H, Pilz S, Scharnagl H, et al. (2008) Independent association of low serum 25-hydroxyvitamin D and 1,25-dihydroxyvitamin D levels with all-cause and cardiovascular mortality. *Arch Intern Med* 168: 1340–1349. http://archinte.jamanetwork.com/article.aspx?articleid=414333
9. Yin K, Agrawal DK. (2014) Vitamin D and inflammatory diseases. *J Inflamm Res* 29(7): 69-87. http://www.ncbi.nlm.nih.gov/pubmed/24971027
10. Huang C, Shapses SA, Wang X. (2013) Association of plasma parathyroid hormone with metabolic syndrome and risk for cardiovascular disease. *Endocr Practice* 19(4): 712-717. http://www.ncbi.nlm.nih.gov/pubmed/23512391
11. van Ballegooijen AJ, Reinders I, Visser M, Brouwer IA. (2013) Parathyroid hormone and cardiovascular disease events: A systematic review and meta-analysis of prospective studies. *Am Heart J* 165(5):655-664. http://www.sciencedirect.com/science/article/pii/S0002870313001415

of fish, which is high in vitamin D, may be protective against coronary heart disease.

But why can't I eat that second slice of cheesecake if my lipids are perfect?

The digestion and absorption of fat in the diet is extremely efficient, with greater than 90% of the fat consumed being rapidly absorbed and transported throughout the body for use or for storage in about five-to-six hours after a meal. This high efficiency and high capacity is evolutionary beneficial. And it also explains why your cousin didn't collapse and die on his way home after he went to an "all the steak you can eat" restaurant and ate three 21-ounce steaks. The body can handle this amount of fat occasionally. Large intakes of nutrients, including fat, occurred throughout history when hunter-gatherers made big kills of animals after times of relatively low food availability.

Overflow of fatty acids in the post-prandial state (after a meal) – the work of Dr. Elizabeth Parks

We now realize that very high amounts of saturated fatty acids can lead to fatty acid toxicity, which is often the result of damaged mitochondria, the powerhouses of the cell, or possibly altered membranes of the endoplasmic reticulum.[12] Repeated intakes of high fat diets may lead to sick or diminished mitochondria in both smooth muscle cells and in the cardiomyocytes, the main work performing cells in heart muscle.

An example how this might occur has been put forth by Dr. Elizabeth Parks. For the past 10 years Dr. Elizabeth Parks has carried out the most exciting and informative studies on fatty

12. Brookheart RT, Michel CI, Schaffer JE. (2009) As a matter of fat. *Cell Metab* 10(1): 9-12. http://www.sciencedirect.com/science/article/pii/S1550413109000898

acid metabolism in humans.[13] She showed how both dietary and stored fat contribute to the free fatty acids that permeate throughout our bodies at every second of the day. Most recently she has documented fatty acid spillover after meals containing fat. The figure below shows how fat is normally absorbed from the small intestine into the blood and how it is then distributed throughout the body for storage or use.

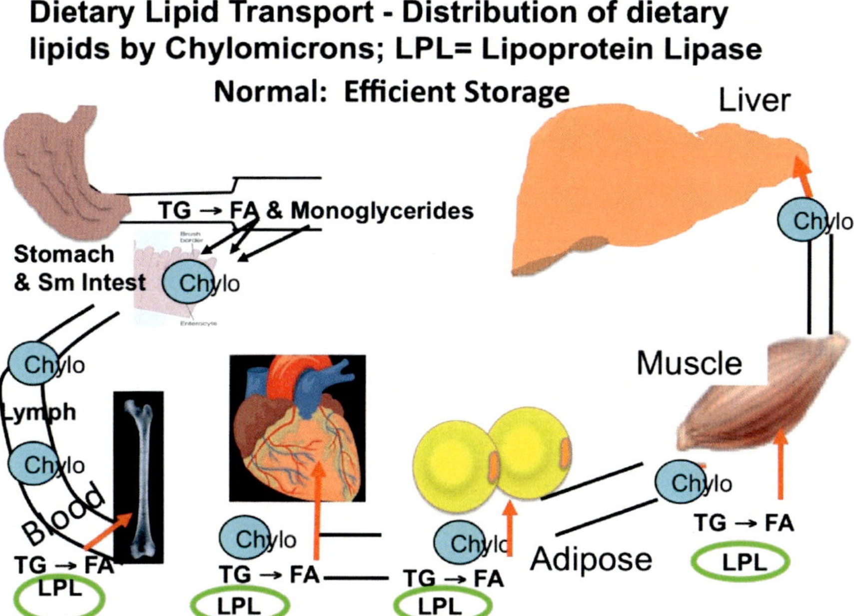

Absorption of dietary lipids and their transport throughout the body on the intestinal derived lipoprotein particle, chylomicron (Chylo). Under normal conditions dietary lipids are absorbed and efficiently transported into tissues. Lipoprotein lipase (LPL) is an enzyme located on the surface of blood vessels and both catches the chylomicron and hydrolyzes the triglyceride (TG) molecules to free fatty acids (FA). Diagram by JL Dixon.

13. Lambert JE, Parks EJ. (2012) Postprandial metabolism of meal triglyceride in humans. *Biochim Biophys Acta.* 1821(5): 721-726 http://www.ncbi.nlm.nih.gov/pmc/articles/PMC3588585/

Fat is digested in the small intestine and is taken up by intestinal cells and packaged into a special lipoprotein called a chylomicron (Chylo).[14 15] Chylomicrons are secreted by intestinal cells into the lymph vessels in the intestine. Chylomicrons are transported in the lymph and are dumped into the blood at the thoracic duct. Once the chylomicrons enter the blood they travel among peripheral tissues where an enzyme, called lipoprotein lipase (LPL in the figures), which is on the surface of the vessels, traps the chylomicrons and causes hydrolysis of the triglycerides to free fatty acids.[16]

Lipoprotein lipase is an integral component of the lipid transportation system in the body. Lipoprotein lipase is a protein/enzyme that is largely attached to the endothelial cells on the side facing the lumen of the artery where it serves as both a dock for chylomicrons and VLDL in the blood and an enzyme that burrows into the cores of lipoproteins and hydrolyzes triglycerides to free fatty acids, which can then enter the cells of tissues. Dr. John Brunzell, of the Department of Medicine, University of Washington, Seattle, spent his long medical career studying lipoprotein lipase and helped a multitude of patients who presented with metabolic problems involving defects in lipoprotein lipase. Very early, Dr. Brunzell investigated the effects of obesity and diabetes on the function of lipoprotein lipase.[17]

14. Hussain MM. (2014) Intestinal lipid absorption and lipoprotein formation. *Curr Opin Lipidol.* 25(3): 200-206. http://www.ncbi.nlm.nih.gov/pubmed/24751933
15. Hussain MM. (2014) Regulation of intestinal lipid absorption by clock genes. *Annu Rev Nutr* 34: 357-375.http://www.annualreviews.org/doi/pdf/10.1146/annurev-nutr-071813-105322
16. Kersten S. (2014) Physiological regulation of lipoprotein lipase. *Biochim Biophys Acta* 1841(7): 919-933. http://www.sciencedirect.com/science/article/pii/S1388198114000663#
17. Pykälistö OJ, Smith PH, Brunzell JD. (1975) Determinants of human adipose tissue lipoprotein lipase. Effect of diabetes and obesity on basal- and diet-induced activity. *J Clin Invest* 56(5): 1108-1117. http://www.jci.org/articles/view/108185

Dr. Brunzell discovered that the high insulin levels observed in obesity increased lipoprotein lipase activity, and that lack of insulin or insulin activity in diabetes decreased lipoprotein lipase activity and increased the risk of hypertriglyceridemia (high blood triglycerides) in diabetes. In 2014, Dr. Brunzell updated his chapter that addressed the treatment of Familial lipoprotein lipase deficiency, a disease that causes severe hypertriglyceridemia.[18] Dr. John Bunzell (Dr. Brunzell passed away in February 2015) was a superb scientist and clinician who helped thousands of patients afflicted with dysregulation of lipid and lipoprotein metabolism.

Through a mechanism that is not even remotely understood, fatty acids that are liberated from triglycerides in lipoproteins enter the various tissues, where they are used for energy (bone marrow, muscle) or where they are stored (adipose tissue, aka fat cells). After permeating through the body, whatever is left of a chylomicron particle is taken up by the liver. The most amazing thing about this process is its efficiency and speed; the half-life of a chylomicron particle once it enters the blood is approximately five minutes.[19]

The second figure depicts a situation where there are much greater numbers of chylomicron particles in the blood and the tissues are not processing the fat fast enough. Therefore, there is fatty acid (FA) spillover into the blood and the fatty acids go to both the liver and the heart. The heart mainly uses fatty acids for energy, but it doesn't have the ability to store large amounts of fat. Therefore, excess fatty acids cause damage to the

18. Brunzell JD. (2014) "Familial Lipoprotein Lipase Deficiency" In: Pagon RA, Adam MP, Ardinger HH, Bird TD, Dolan CR, Fong CT, Smith RJH, Stephens K, editors. Gene Reviews® 1993-2014 [Internet]. Seattle (WA): University of Washington, Seattle [updated 2014 Apr 24]. http://www.ncbi.nlm.nih.gov/books/NBK1308/
19. Park Y, Damron BD, Miles JM, Harris WS. (2001) Measurement of human chylomicron triglyceride clearance with a labeled commercial lipid emulsion. *Lipids* 36(2):115-120. http://link.springer.com/article/10.1007/s11745-001-0696-6

mitochondria and other organelles of the heart cells. The damage is probably not significant in the short term, but after many years of this abuse, there can be loss of active cardiomyocytes, the workhorses of the heart. Proliferation of heart smooth muscle cells also occurs and can cause plaque growth.

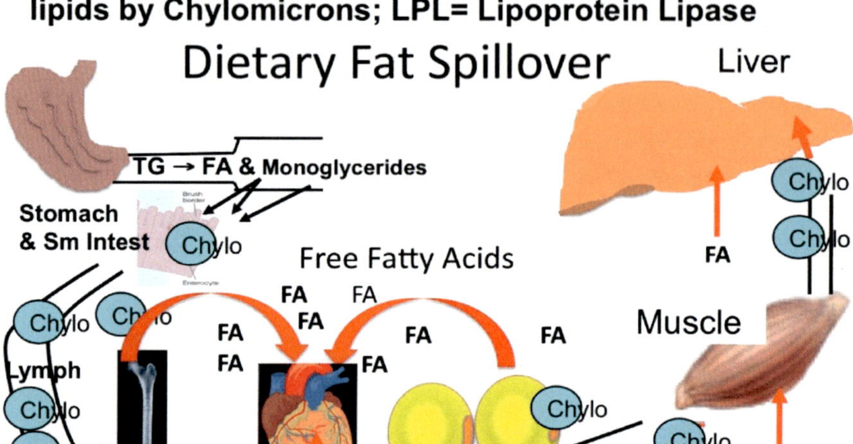

Absorption of dietary lipids under abnormal conditions. The diagram depicts the transport of dietary lipids throughout the body on chylomicrons (Chylo) when a large amount of fat is consumed. In the depicted scenario, the increased number of chylomicron particles overwhelm the uptake mechanism and, therefore, free fatty acids (FA) are released and taken up by the heart cardiomyocytes and smooth muscle cells, which can be damaged by very high levels of fatty acids. Diagram by JL Dixon.

Dietary fat that is transported into the blood has to be efficiently stored in adipose or rapidly oxidized in peripheral tissues like muscle. If not, there will be spillover into the free fatty acid pool in blood and this could make its way to the heart. Conditions that exacerbate the spillover are lack of exercise, diabetes, and very large fat meals.[20] So in addition to bringing in those extra Kcal, that second piece of cheesecake provides extra fatty acids that may damage your heart mitochondria or cause plaque buildup.

The blood lipids that your doctor measures are levels of lipids that are in your blood in the fasting state (usually in the morning before breakfast). But all of what I described above happens after you eat a meal. Therefore, your fasting blood lipids can be perfect, but you may be doing yourself harm by consistently eating a high-saturated-fat diet.

Remember, humans needed to process huge amounts of fat after that successful hunt, so occasionally, it is okay to eat that first piece of cheesecake or to enjoy Thanksgiving dinner with friends and family.

20. Jacome-Sosa MM, Parks EJ. (2014) Fatty acid sources and their fluxes as they contribute to plasma triglyceride concentrations and fatty liver in humans. *Curr Opin Lipidol* 25(3): 213-220. http://www.ncbi.nlm.nih.gov/pubmed/?term=24785962

PART III.

LIVING THE MEDITERRANEAN WAY

15.

LIVING THE MEDITERRANEAN WAY: DISCOVERY OF THE MEDITERRANEAN DIET

In 1962 Dr. Keys and his family moved to Pioppi, Italy, a small fishing village about a four hour drive south of the city of Naples. The house they finally settled in is on the Cilento coast and overlooks the Mediterranean Sea, and Dr. Keys named it "Minnelea," from the first letters of Minnesota and the ancient Greek Elea. Quite remarkably, houses in the same grouping where the Keyses lived can be rented during the summer months by contacting Mr. Armando Troccoli. The image below is a view of the Cilento coast very close to Pioppi, Italy. The second image shows a Mediterranean meal ready to be consumed.

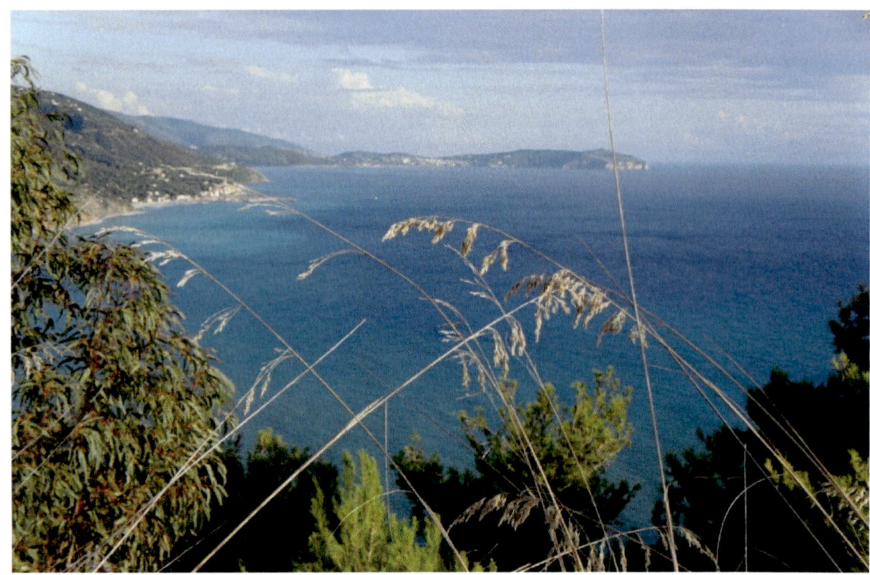

View of the Cilento coast. Photo used by permission of Armando Troccoli (www.cilento.de).

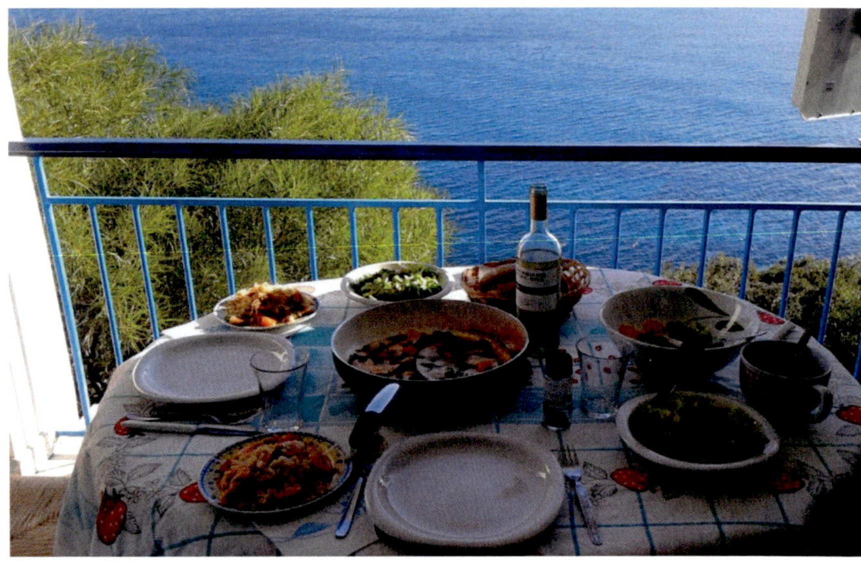

Mediterranean meal overlooking the shore of the Cilento coast. Photograph used by permission of Armando Troccoli (www.cilento.de).

Mr. Armando Troccoli is a native of the Cilento and grew up near Pioppi and commented the following to me:[1]

> I live here in the Cilento. Was born here in a small village called Terradura. Very close Velia. With a view to the sea and the village Pioppi. Here lived Dr. Ancel Keys, his wife and his friends ... I believe that few residents have understood [during] his lifetime, what Dr. Keys was concerned ... as always in life, you feel later is what scientists of "Keys" has explored ... Today, the people here are proud of the work and discoveries. "The mediterranean diet" was created thanks to Dr. Keys. The UNESCO has recognized this and as the "Dieta Mediterranea" with the properties that Ancel Keys had recognized and researched on the spot, the best, therefore, recognized as the healthiest diet.

What was the Mediterranean diet like when the Seven Countries Study was just underway? What was the "Mediterranean diet" as Dr. Keys observed it?

In Chapter 2 of their book, *How to Eat Well and Stay Well the Mediterranean Way,*[2] Dr. Keys and Margaret wrote about the foods they found in the Mediterranean countries they visited and the Mediterranean lifestyle they observed in their travels. They made the comment in the beginning of the Chapter that they were specifically talking about the countries of Greece, Italy, the Mediterranean portion of France, and Spain. Each had their own special dishes and customs. The location they knew best was southern Italy, because they had decided to move to a house in southern Italy for at least six months of the year while Dr. Keys

1. Communication with Armando Troccoli on February 22, 2015. Mr. Troccoli's address is: Piazza dell'Unione 14 84070 TERRADURA (SA), and his website is: www.cilento.de
2. *Keys A, Keys M. (1975) How to Eat Well and Stay Well the Mediterranean Way.* Garden City, New York: Doubleday & Company

was still working, and for almost the full year after he retired in 1972.

What was the Mediterranean diet the Keyses observed and experienced?

Vegetables and fruits.

The availability of vegetables and fruits depended upon the season. Early in the spring there were cauliflower, artichokes, and lettuce available. Later, there were fava beans and a dozen different wild greens in the markets of their fishing village. Later still came spinach, green beans, and zucchini. Late spring brought cherries, kumquats, and mushrooms.

Summer brought figs, tomatoes, eggplants, peppers, and onions. At the end of summer, wine was prepared during the grape harvest. All sorts of melons were available in the early fall. From their own property they harvested apples, pears, and a whole family of citrus fruits. Late fall saw the production of persimmons, pomegranates, and finally olives. In the end, one senses that there was a cornucopia of fresh vegetables and fruits that they were exposed to from the local farms and hillsides all year round.

Olives.

Olives pressed early in the season were the source of virgin olive oil. A small percentage of olives were prepared for whole storage to be used as table olives during the year. The largest per capita consumption of olive oil occurred on Crete, where it provided 30% of the total caloric intake. In other areas of the Mediterranean, olive oil provided from 15% to 20% of total calories. French cooking used more butter and therefore was not as healthy as the cuisines of Greece and Italy.

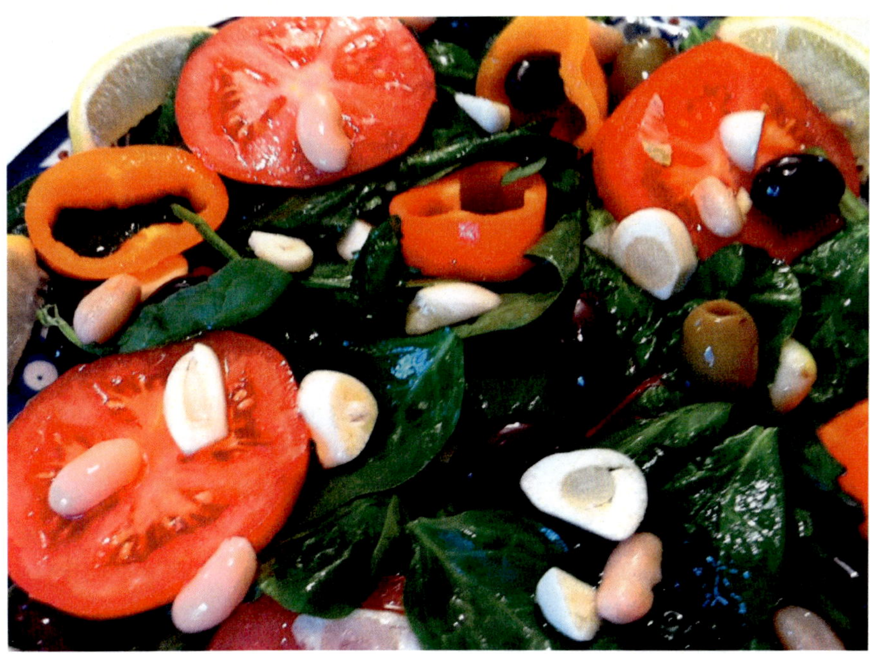

Mediterranean lunch. Prepared and photographed by Marlene Perchinske.

Bread.

Freshly baked bread provided a considerable amount of calories for diverse populations in the Mediterranean region. In Greece, it could provide up to 38% of the total calories consumed. In other countries it was less, but it still was a significant percentage of the total calories consumed. On average, at the time of Dr. Keys's investigations, three times more bread was eaten in the Mediterranean areas compared to what was eaten in the United States.

Dessert.

Fruit was the main dessert served in Mediterranean households. Sweet desserts were reserved for holidays. Peoples of the

Mediterranean region ate, on average, 150% more fruit than Americans.

Garlic and onions.

These were used in cooking, stews, and salads. Garlic soup is a specialty of the Spanish, whereas the French are known for their onion soup. The Italians are known for their *bruschetta*, which is a slice of hot toast brushed with olive oil and raw garlic.

Tomatoes and garden greens.

Mediterraneans harvested tomatoes and prepared homemade tomato sauce every August. Bottled tomato sauce was used throughout the year in stews and with pastas. Also eaten all year round was a vast array of leafy greens that come from the garden or from the roadside. The Mediterranean peoples ate a much wider variety of greens than do Americans.

Dr. Keys wrote in a later article, "Near our second home in southern Italy, all kinds of leaves are an important part of the everyday diet. There are many kinds of lettuce, spinach, Swiss chard, purslane, and plants I cannot identify with an English name such as *lettuga, barbabietole, scarola,* and *rape*. Some are perennials. The climate permits replanting annuals several times a year so leaves to eat are always at hand. No main meal in the Mediterranean countries is replete without lots of dure (greens). *Mangiafoglia* is the Italian word for "to eat leaves" and that is a key part of the good Mediterranean diet."[3]

3. Keys A. (1995) Mediterranean diet and public health: personal reflections. *Am J Clin Nutr* 61(6 Suppl): 1321S-1323S. http://www.ncbi.nlm.nih.gov/pubmed/?term=7754982

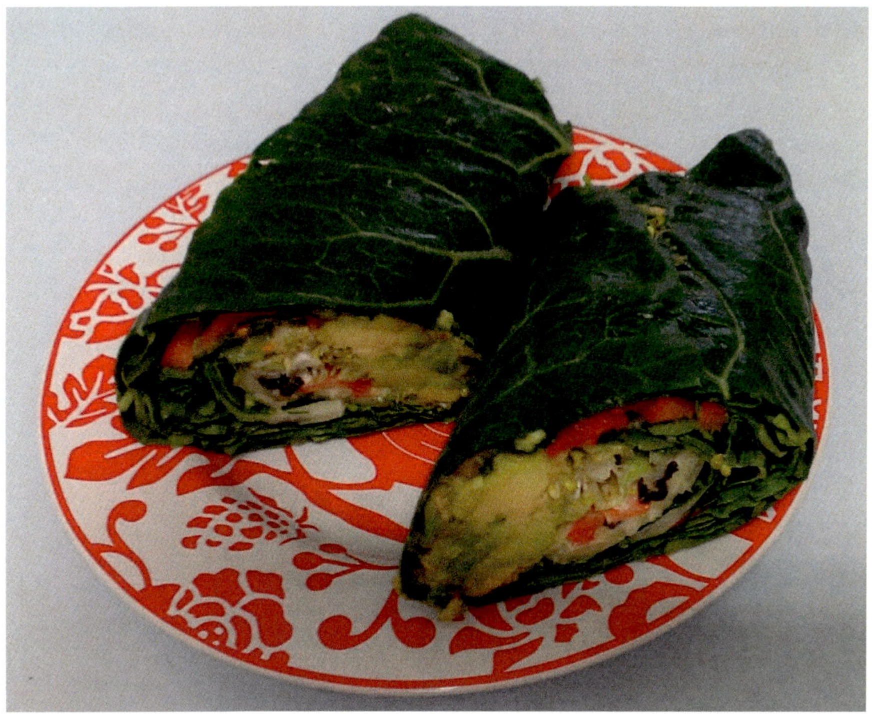

Collards green wrap–certainly healthier than a hamburger! Prepared by Marlene Perchinske and Sharon Jacques. Photograph by Sharon Jacques.

Seafood and Meat.

Inhabitants of the Mediterranean region were strong consumers of anchovies, octopus, mackerel, dried codfish from northern seas, and a vast array of ocean fish. Fish caught directly from the Mediterranean Sea were less plentiful because the Mediterranean had been overfished at this time.

Americans were eating four times more meat than what was consumed in Greece and Spain. In Mediterranean countries more veal was consumed than beef, except in France. Only about half the eggs Americans ate were consumed by Mediterraneans. The French ate more butter than Americans, but the other

Mediterranean countries consumed only about one third to one half the butter Americans did at the time.

Beverages.

The consumption of wine was much greater in Mediterranean countries, but it was usually consumed with main meals. For men, the amount of wine consumed possibly amounted to about 10% of total caloric intake coming from alcohol. There was very little consumption of hard liquor except on special occasions.

The Mediterranean people are known to drink strong and freshly made coffee, often using an "espresso" machine. In fact, coffee with added hot milk was a common breakfast for them. Spain was the one country where people also drank a considerable amount of hot cocoa. Other drinks that were popular were lemonade, cola drinks, and mineral water. Cola drinks were not consumed at the level consumed in the United States at the time.

The Intangibles.

Mediterraneans were more likely to take an evening stroll than Americans. They were also likely to eat a wider variety of foods, especially fresh seafood and vegetables. Because of the southern sun, they received more sunlight on a yearly basis, spread more evenly throughout the year, than in northern regions where people are subjected to periods of little sun during winter, followed by intense sun exposure during the summer. The climate allowed for a longer and more consistent period of moderate vitamin D availability (due to formation of vitamin D in the skin in response to sunlight) in the Mediterranean region.

At the time Dr. Ancel Keys and Margaret wrote their Mediterranean cookbook, they noted that although the expenditures of the Mediterranean countries on health care were much less than that expended in the United States, the Mediterraneans' "overall health and longevity are impressive, both in the vital statistics and in our own many years of scientific observations."[4]

The main difference in health was that there was a much lower rate of coronary heart disease in Mediterranean countries compared to the United States. Dr. Keys specifically commented that, from his vast experience in the region, the difference was not explained by climate, genes, nor the way disease was diagnosed nor how statistics were kept in the different countries. And another plus was that deaths from all causes were lower in the Mediterranean countries than in the United States.

The remainder of the book, *How to Eat Well and Stay Well the Mediterranean Way*, is chock full of health information and recipes of all types, and as stated by the Keyses in the authors' preface, all were tested first in their kitchens, sometimes in Pioppi, Italy, sometimes in Minnesota, before they were entered into their cookbook.

Their book was the first one to promote the Mediterranean diet. Combined with the early chapters on diet and health, it represents an additional major triumph in the life of this extraordinary scientist and his companion spouse.

An Example of a Mediterranean Diet over the course of a day

Today the Mediterranean diet is as easy to follow in the United States as the Keyses practiced it in their village on the coast of Italy. Most of the ingredients are available the year round in the markets of major cities. Below is the summary of the meals from a day's menu that follows the Mediterranean diet. This summary was produced using the excellent United States Department of Agriculture SuperTracker Website that relies on the most comprehensive food composition tables available.[5]

4. Keys A, Keys M. (1975) *How to Eat Well and Stay Well the Mediterranean Way.* Garden City, New York: Doubleday & Company. page 42.
5. United States Department of Agriculture. https://www.supertracker.usda.gov/default.aspx

USDA Meals Summary for a Mediterranean Diet with Extra Protein

Breakfast	Lunch	Dinner	Snacks
• ¾ cup, cut stalks Broccoli, fresh, cooked (no salt or fat added)	• 1 small breast Chicken, breast, boneless, skinless, grilled	• 1 tablespoon Almonds, chocolate covered	• 1 medium (7" to 7-7/8" long) Banana, raw
• ¼ cup, shredded Cheese, Mozzarella, part skim	• ¼ cup Chickpeas (garbanzo beans), canned (no fat added)	• ½ cup, slices Beets, fresh, cooked (no salt or fat added)	
• 2 mug (8 fl oz) Coffee, brewed, regular	• ¼ cup, sliced Cucumber, raw	• 1 medium scoop Frozen yogurt, vanilla, low fat	
• 2 large egg white Egg whites, cooked, no fat added	• 1 tablespoon, crumbled Feta cheese	• 2 tablespoon Oil, olive	
• ½ tablespoon Half and half	• ½ cup, chopped Kale, raw	• 1 cup Rice, brown, regular, cooked (no salt or fat added)	
• 3 teaspoon Oil, olive	• 1 cup Milk, low fat (1%)	• 1 medium fillet Salmon, baked or broiled, with oil	
• ¼ cup Onion, fresh, cooked (no salt or fat added)	• ¼ cup, sliced or chopped Olives, green	• ¾ cup, slices Squash, summer (yellow or zucchini), fresh, cooked (no salt or fat added)	
• 1 cup Orange juice, carton, can, or bottle	• 1 medium (2-5/8" across) Orange, raw	• 3 piece Sushi, with vegetables, rolled in seaweed	
• 1 medium (2-5/8" across) Orange, raw	• ½ package (10 oz) Spinach, raw		
• ½ cup, chopped or sliced Tomato, raw	• 1 tablespoon Vinegar, balsamic		

Highlights:
High Fiber
High Potassium
High Vitamin K
High Folate
Emphasizes:
High Monounsaturated Fat
Low Saturated Fat
High Omega-3 Fatty Acids

Summary of meals from one day of the Mediterranean Diet. Generated using the USDA SuperTracker Website. United States Department of Agriculture; https://www.supertracker.usda.gov/default.aspx

The keys to this diet are using fresh vegetables, including different types of greens, olive oil for cooking, and protein sources with low saturated fat. This particular diet example illustrates the use of high protein sources because the author prefers to eat like this. Using the above meals as a template, it is easy to make substitutions with similar type foods so that the diet does not become monotonous. One characteristic of the Mediterranean diet is that it does not include processed foods, a main source of sodium in the diet. The USDA Supertracker Website provided the nutrient analysis for this day. The program lists the target daily nutrients (based upon the Recommended Daily Allowances (RDAs) or other Dietary Reference Intakes-see Nutrition.gov)[6] appropriate for the profile that the user submits to the Website–in this case, a fairly active 35-year old male.

Daily Nutrients Supplied by the Mediterranean Diet with Extra Protein

Nutrients 35-Year Old Male:	Target	Average Eaten	Status
⊞ Total Calories	2400 Calories	2385 Calories	OK
⊞ Protein (g)***	56 g	150 g ←	OK
⊞ Protein (% Calories)***	10 - 35% Calories	25% Calories ←	OK
⊞ Carbohydrate (g)***	130 g	248 g	OK
⊞ Carbohydrate (% Calories)***	45 - 65% Calories	42% Calories	Under
⊞ Dietary Fiber	38 g	33 g ←	Under
⊞ Total Sugars	No Daily Target or Limit	123 g	No Daily Target or Limit
⊞ Added Sugars	No Daily Target or Limit	17 g	No Daily Target or Limit
⊞ Total Fat	20 - 35% Calories	35% Calories ←	OK
⊞ Saturated Fat	< 10% Calories	7% Calories ←	OK
⊞ Polyunsaturated Fat	No Daily Target or Limit	7% Calories	No Daily Target or Limit
⊞ Monounsaturated Fat	No Daily Target or Limit	18% Calories	No Daily Target or Limit
⊞ Linoleic Acid (g)***	17 g	12 g	Under
⊞ Linoleic Acid (% Calories)***	5 - 10% Calories	4% Calories	Under
⊞ α-Linolenic Acid (% Calories)***	0.6 - 1.2% Calories	0.7% Calories	OK
⊞ α-Linolenic Acid (g)***	1.6 g	1.8 g	OK
⊞ Omega 3 - EPA	No Daily Target or Limit	1413 mg ←	No Daily Target or Limit
⊞ Omega 3 - DHA	No Daily Target or Limit	1980 mg	No Daily Target or Limit
⊞ Cholesterol	< 300 mg	282 mg ←	OK

← = Highlight

Daily Macronutrients Supplied by the Mediterranean Diet with Slightly Higher Protein Intake. Generated using the United States Department of Agriculture SuperTracker Website.

Daily Nutrients Supplied by the Mediterranean Diet with Extra Protein

Minerals 35-Year Old Male:	Target	Average Eaten	Status
⊞ Calcium	1000 mg	1334 mg ←	OK
⊞ Potassium	4700 mg	6074 mg ←	OK
⊞ Sodium**	< 2300 mg	2992 mg ←	Over
⊞ Copper	900 µg	2268 µg	OK
⊞ Iron	8 mg	15 mg	OK
⊞ Magnesium	420 mg	629 mg	OK
⊞ Phosphorus	700 mg	2220 mg	OK
⊞ Selenium	55 µg	234 µg	OK
⊞ Zinc	11 mg	11 mg	OK

Daily Minerals Supplied by the Mediterranean Diet with Slightly Higher Protein Intake.

6. http://www.nutrition.gov/smart-nutrition-101/dietary-reference-intakes-rdas

Daily Nutrients Supplied by the Mediterranean Diet with Extra Protein

Vitamins	35-Year Old Male: Target	Average Eaten	Status
⊞ Vitamin A	900 µg RAE	1353 µg RAE	OK
⊞ Vitamin B6	1.3 mg	3.4 mg	OK
⊞ Vitamin B12	2.4 µg	10.3 µg ←	OK
⊞ Vitamin C	90 mg	422 mg	OK
⊞ Vitamin D	15 µg	29 µg ←	OK
⊞ Vitamin E	15 mg AT	20 mg AT	OK
⊞ Vitamin K	120 µg	1144 µg ←	OK
⊞ Folate	400 µg DFE	847 µg DFE ←	OK
⊞ Thiamin	1.2 mg	1.9 mg	OK
⊞ Riboflavin	1.3 mg	2.8 mg	OK
⊞ Niacin	16 mg	45 mg	OK
⊞ Choline	550 mg	657 mg	OK

Daily Vitamins Supplied by the Mediterranean Diet with Slightly Higher Protein Intake.

The red arrows indicate the highlights of the Mediterranean diet. The protein content of the example was fairly high as it represented 25% of total Kcal intake. This is a personal preference as eating a higher protein diet feels right for the author. The dietary fiber was 33 grams, which is slightly below the recommended amount. This illustrates how difficult it is to obtain enough fiber because one would expect by scanning the meal summary that this particular diet would have sufficient fiber. Total fat was 35% of total Kcal intake, and the saturated fat was only 7% of total Kcal in the diet. The omega-3 fatty acid intake was moderate with total amounts of omega-3 fatty acids adding up to above 3 grams per day. This is largely the result of the salmon consumed this particular day. The cholesterol content of the diet was below 300 mg. This level was attained by using egg whites instead of whole eggs for breakfast. This very simple manipulation eliminated 200 mg of cholesterol from the day's intake. Carbohydrate represented about 40% of total Kcal intake. This amount is neither very high nor very low, and simple sugars only made up 14% of total carbohydrates in the diet. Linoleic and alpha-linolenic acids were slightly low, but most authorities would consider the high intake of omega-3 fatty acids as adequate compensation.

The intake of minerals was extremely good across the board. Potassium intake was more than adequate. An intake of 6,074 mg of potassium is a result of consumption of fresh fruits and vegetables. Calcium intake was extremely strong. Sodium intake was identified as being over the target level because the target level of <2,300 mg for a 35-year old male is set extremely low. However, the level of sodium (2,992 mg) in this diet was quite reasonable. If you have high blood pressure, you will certainly wish to pay closer attention to the sodium content of your diet. All the other minerals were safely above the target levels.

All the vitamins in the diet were sufficient, and the levels of four vitamins were probably the greatest highlight of this diet–vitamin B12, vitamin D, vitamin K, and folate were 429, 193, 953, and 212% of the target levels. These four vitamins are very high in the Mediterranean diet, and it has been proposed that these vitamins are especially important in maintaining health–especially in older adults. Therefore, the Mediterranean diet is excellent at protecting against coronary heart disease throughout life, and it is also capable of protecting cognitive function during the twilight years.

16.

WHAT WE KNOW ABOUT THE MEDITERRANEAN DIET TODAY

If you read *How to Eat Well and Stay Well the Mediterranean Way,*[1] published in 1975 and a *New York Times* best seller, you will recognize that Dr. Ancel Keys and Margaret Keys wrote an expansive review of diet and health that quite frankly cannot be surpassed by later cookbooks by other authors. This is my opinion, but I hope someday the book will become available again so that you get the chance to read it. The vast amount of information in the book is staggering, and the recipes are real and every one of them was tested by the Keys family in their own kitchen.

Prior to *How to Eat Well and Stay Well the Mediterranean Way,* the Keyses had written and published in 1959, *Eat Well and Stay Well.*[2] The first section of this book is entitled "Diet and Health" and focuses on classical basic nutrition including the

1. Keys A, Keys M. (1975) How to Eat Well and Stay Well the Mediterranean Way. Garden City, New York: Doubleday & Company.
2. Keys A, Keys M. (1959) *Eat Well and Stay Well.* Garden City, New York: Doubleday & Company.

macronutrients and the energy content of foods. It also discusses the role of exercise in maintaining body weight. Section two gives basic information about specific foods and how to cook them. Section three includes a four week menu that can be used to eat healthy and reduce Kcal intake. Section four provides over a hundred pages of recipes. The recipes that the Keyses included in this book are largely derived from the meals they observed on their multiple trips to the Mediterranean area during the Seven Countries Study.

Having read the three cookbooks that the Keyses wrote, the misinformation concerning Dr. Keys and his views on nutrition and health that is promulgated by some media personalities today is hard to explain. One wonders whether they have taken the time to read Dr. Keys's scientific writings, including *Seven Countries,* the monographs, the hundreds of scientific articles, and the three cookbooks that Dr. Keys and Margaret Keys wrote.

Dr. Keys spent most of his career studying physiology, nutrition, and health. And during a very long career, he made many discoveries, including these major accomplishments that have had a great impact on the American people:

1. He formulated ready-to-eat meals (called K-rations) for the American armed forces during World War II. These turned out to be a technical success and are immortalized in hundreds of movies and books about World War II.

2. He led a major study during World War II on starvation that provided important information on how to treat starved prisoners and civilians.

3. He conceived and implemented the Seven Countries Study and identified important dietary factors that were associated with coronary heart disease.

4. He led a series of controlled dietary fat and cholesterol feeding studies in humans that resulted in the "Keys Equation," which accurately predicted the changes in blood cholesterol

concentrations when changes were made in the composition of fats in the diet.

But in my opinion, the true genius of Dr. Keys was displayed when he and Margaret Keys wrote their three cookbooks, including the 470-page cookbook, *How to Eat Well and Stay Well the Mediterranean Way*. This book clearly explained the effects of diet on health and disease, and then it went on to show how to prepare healthy Mediterranean meals through the tested recipes in the book. It was their attempt to disseminate their knowledge directly to the American public, and they were successful to some extent because their books ended up on the *New York Times* best sellers list. However, the problem in all this was that the message did not get out to everyone. And when the books went out of print, they were no longer available to provide guidance to Americans. So later generations were not helped by their cookbooks.

Quite honestly, I never heard of *How to Eat Well and Stay Well the Mediterranean Way* before I started to write about Ancel Keys. In fact, as I discussed earlier, it was difficult to find the book. And when I read it, I was absolutely amazed at the vast amount of information that it conveyed. The most surprising observations in the entire book were that Dr. Keys stated conclusively that total fat intake was not the most important and dominant factor in the development of coronary heart disease. On the contrary, it was clearly written that the type of dietary fat was the most important factor in its development. This conclusion came from his accumulated experiences studying the diet-cholesterol-coronary heart disease connection for a large part of his career. It was most clearly delineated when he visited Crete and observed that although the total fat Kcal consumed on Crete was very high, there was essentially zero coronary heart disease on the island. Dr. Keys scoured the island and could not find any patients with coronary heart disease in hospitals or being treated by doctors.

This was especially important in convincing Dr. Keys that total fat was not the main culprit in coronary heart disease.

How to Eat Well and Stay Well the Mediterranean Way was published in 1975 and *Seven Countries* was published in 1980, and, unfortunately, there was very little overlap in the background material that was presented in each book. This may have been a mistake in strategy, because anyone who did not read *How to Eat Well and Stay Well the Mediterranean Way,* because it was a cookbook, missed out on a wealth of information that it conveyed about how the Seven Countries Study was started and carried out. And likewise, people who just read the cookbook were not able to appreciate the vast amount of data collected in all 16 cohorts of the Seven Countries Study. But somehow the messages that Dr. Keys and Margaret clearly wrote about were short lived, and because of this, some of the conclusions reached by Dr. Keys were needlessly debated by researchers in the cardiovascular field for many years afterward.

But today, news about the Mediterranean diet is being spread by a whole new crop of researchers and physicians. Even recently, a study[3] was published in 2013 on the Mediterranean diet that supported most of the early observations of Dr. Keys.

This study on the protective effects of the Mediterranean diet on coronary heart disease was called the PREDIMED Study and was conducted by Dr. Ramon Estruch of the University of Barcelona along with other researchers from throughout Spain. It was a dietary intervention trial that was designed to have three groups: a control group that was instructed on how to eat a conventional low-fat diet; and two groups that were instructed on how to eat a Mediterranean diet, with increased olive oil intake the cornerstone of one group, and increased intake of a mixture of nuts the cornerstone of the other group. When the study was

3. Estruch R. *et al.* (PREDIMED Study Investigators) (2013) Primary prevention of cardiovascular disease with a Mediterranean diet. *New England Journal of Medicine* 368(14): 1279-1290. http://www.nejm.org/doi/full/10.1056/NEJMoa1200303

published in the *New England Journal of Medicine* in April 2013, it raised a great deal of discussion in the nutrition field due to its findings and experimental design.

The most important observation made in the study was that even when participants (with no cardiovascular disease at enrollment) were recruited quite late in life (men – 55 to 80 years of age; and women – 60 to 80 years of age), a traditional Mediterranean diet with either ample intake of olive oil or ample intake of nuts was protective (a relative risk reduction of approximately 30%) against major cardiovascular events (acute myocardial infarction, stroke, or death from cardiovascular causes) when all three were analyzed together versus the recommended conventional low-fat diet that the control group was instructed to consume.

As in all large studies with humans, there were problems with this study. As pointed out by Dr. Dean Ornish in a letter to the editor of *New England Journal of Medicine*,[4] the diet the control participants actually consumed was a high-fat diet, with 37% of the Kcal coming from fat. Another criticism of the study was that, when each category was analyzed individually, only the stroke category was significantly decreased in the groups consuming the two prescribed Mediterranean diets.

Also, there was something missing in the discussion section of the Estruch study, and this was the acknowledgment that the results largely supported the observations that Dr. Keys and his colleagues had made much earlier in the Seven Countries Study.

However, the editors of the *New England Journal of Medicine* asked Dr. Sarah Tracy, an historian of science, to write an editorial[5] to connect the 2013 PREDIMED Study article to earlier

4. Ornish D. (2013) Mediterranean Diet for Primary Prevention of Cardiovascular Disease. *N Engl J Med* 369: 672-677. August 15, 2013 http://www.nejm.org/doi/full/10.1056/NEJMoa1200303#t=letters
5. Tracy SW. (2013) Something New Under the Sun? The Mediterranean Diet and Cardiovascular Health. *N Engl J Med* 368(14): 1274-1276. http://www.nejm.org/doi/full/10.1056/NEJMp1302616

work by Dr. Keys and the many other scientists who contributed to the Seven Countries Study.

Dr. Tracy wrote:

> The first epidemiologic data supporting the Mediterranean diet came from the Seven Countries Study (SCS), a prospective investigation of diet and other cardiovascular-disease risk factors in 16 cohorts totaling nearly 13,000 men in the United States, Italy, Greece, Yugoslavia, Finland, the Netherlands, and Japan, which began in 1958.....The PREDIMED results would come as little surprise to the man behind the SCS, American physiologist and epidemiologist Ancel Keys, who advanced the low-fat diet and the low-saturated fat Mediterranean diet for the primary and secondary prevention of heart disease. Keys "discovered" the Mediterranean diet's health benefits in the early 1950s, when visiting the region as a medical scientist concerned about the widely reported increase in heart attacks in the United States.

In my mind, the Estruch study from Spain was an important study because it showed the protective effects of the Mediterranean diet after a relatively short period of time. The most amazing outcome of the study was that the protective effects of the Mediterranean diet were observed in an older population after only approximately five years of implementation. In fact, the study was stopped after a median follow-up of 4.8 years because the results were so persuasive, and the investigators thought it was not ethical to continue the control population, which had higher rates of cardiovascular disease, on the prescribed control diet.

Interestingly, there was one major difference between the results observed in Dr. Estruch's study compared to the earlier results observed by Dr. Keys. This was that in the Estruch study, there were no differences in the rates of total deaths from all causes between the populations consuming the Mediterranean diet and the control population that was consuming the control diet. In contrast, at the time of Ancel Keys's Seven Countries

Study, there were in fact lower total death rates (from all causes) in populations who consumed a Mediterranean diet compared to the participants in the United States and northern Europe, who consumed a classic Western style diet (See figures below drawn from tables that were in the appendix of *How to Eat Well and Stay Well the Mediterranean Way*).[6]

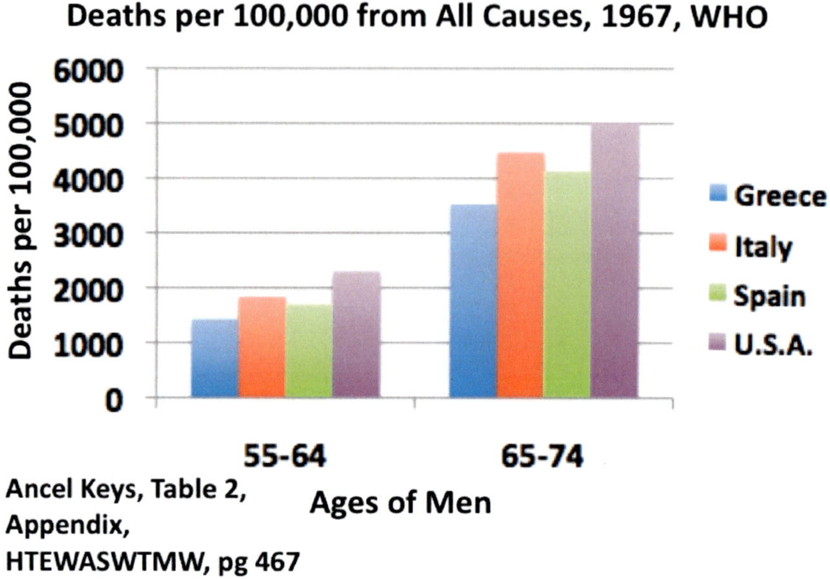

Deaths from All Causes in 1967. Data from the World Health Organization (WHO) that was presented in Table 2 of the appendix of *How to Eat Well and Stay Well the Mediterranean Way*, page 467. Graphed by JL Dixon.

6. Keys A, Keys M. (1975) *How to Eat Well and Stay Well the Mediterranean Way.* Garden City, New York: Doubleday & Company, page 467.

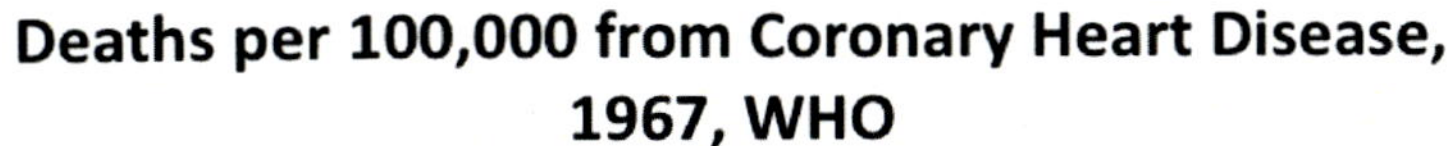

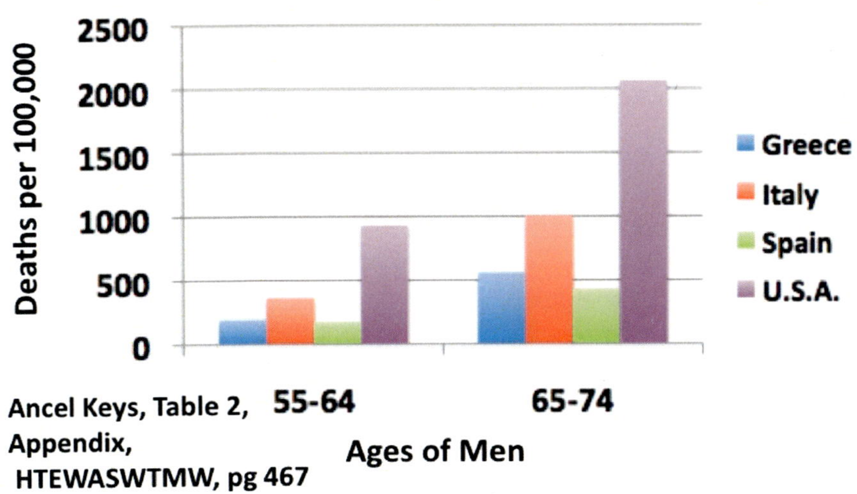

Deaths from Coronary Heart Disease in 1967. Data from the World Health Organization (WHO) that was presented in Table 2 of the appendix of *How to Eat Well and Stay Well the Mediterranean Way*, page 467. Graphed by JL Dixon.

The differences in these important outcomes were probably due to the fact that at the time of Keys's investigations, the populations studied had been consuming the Mediterranean diet for most of their lives, and thus they received more comprehensive protective effects. Also, the populations in the other regions were consuming a higher saturated-fat diet for most of their lives.

Other studies have pointed to the protective effects of the Mediterranean diet. A 2010 meta-analysis, involving more than two million total subjects among all of the examined and included studies, investigated the role of the Mediterranean diet in enhancing heath.[7] The authors developed an adherence scale and

7. Sofi F, Abbate R, Gensini GF, Casini A. (2010) Accruing evidence on benefits

the meta-analysis showed that a two-point increase in adherence to the Mediterranean diet was associated with an 8% reduction of death from all causes, a 10% reduction in incidence of cardio- and cerebrovascular diseases, a 6% reduction in the incidence of neoplastic diseases, and a 13% reduction in the incidence of neurodegenerative diseases. At first reading these reductions do not seem that significant, but one has to remember that in current times, people in many Mediterranean areas are subjected to other factors, such as lower overall physical activity, in addition to food, that promote a more Western lifestyle.

When discussing the utility of the Mediterranean diet in some of these more modern studies, the most important question would be the one that Dr. Ancel Keys would conceivably ask first, "Is the Mediterranean diet that is being proposed today the same Mediterranean diet that he studied in the 1950s, when the coronary heart disease rates were extremely low to nonexistent?" One problem with the more recent studies of the health promoting effects of the Mediterranean diet is that the participants are greatly affected and influenced by Western lifestyle and the media. However, Estruch's study, and the 2010 meta-analysis, show that the positive effects of the Mediterranean diet can still be observed today.

Therefore, a general conclusion is that populations who consume a Mediterranean diet for their entire lives not only exhibit lower rates of cardiovascular disease, but they also live longer, healthier lives, too, compared to populations eating a Western diet along with living a Western lifestyle. But happily, changing to a Mediterranean diet late in life still conveys protective effects.

of adherence to the Mediterranean diet on health: an updated systematic review and meta-analysis. *Am J Clin Nutr* 92(5): 1189-1196. http://ajcn.nutrition.org/content/92/5/1189.long

17.

GENIUS AND PARTNERSHIP

In 1962 Dr. Keys and Margaret moved to Pioppi, Italy, south of the city of Naples. The house they finally built and settled in is on the Cilento coast and overlooks the Mediterranean Sea.

In September 1987, Michael Moore wrote in the University of Minnesota Health Sciences Public Relations quarterly, *Update:* "They purchased the land with friends while visiting Naples from 63-64. The Keys and their four research colleagues built homes and the Keys called it Minnelea."[1] Dr. Keys named it Minnelea, from the first letters of Minnesota and the ancient Greek name Elea. In Dr. Keys's files at the Division of Epidemiology, I found an undated comprehensive history[2] (in Dr. Keys' longhand and also typed, too) of the Greek settlement, Elea, that is located a few miles south of his home in Pioppi: "A few miles south are the remnants of the Greek City, *Elea*, now bearing the Italian name,

1. Moore M. (1987) *Update*. September issue. Quarterly publication of the University of Minnesota.
2. Keys A. History of Elea, Archives of Dr. Ancel Keys and Margaret Keys, and the Seven Countries Study. University of Minnesota Division of Epidemiology and Community Health. Courtesy of Dr. H Blackburn. http://www.epi.umn.edu/cvdepi/

Velia. Greeks settled *Elea* in 535 BC. A few years earlier they had fled from invaders attacking their home on the Turkish coast of the Aegean Sea." This story by Dr. Keys continued on for several pages and gave the thorough history of the village.

Through the late 1980s Dr. Keys continued to work on writing up reports and studies connected to the Seven Countries Study, but he slowed down a little as the decade proceeded due to failing eyesight brought on by macular degeneration.[3]

An international symposium was convened in 1993 to celebrate Dr. Keys's 90th birthday. This symposium, organized by Professor H. Toshimain of Japan, was called "Lessons for Science from the Seven Countries Study" and was held in Fukuoka, Japan. Dr. and Mrs. Keys attended and the participants decided to assemble a history of the Seven Countries Study with all the principal investigators of the cohorts contributing to this endeavor. A monograph was produced that has been referenced throughout this book.[4]

Ancel Keys kept on giving lively and interesting interviews. In 1997 a reporter Peter Jaret, from *Eating Well* magazine,[5] interviewed Dr. Keys when he and Margaret were visiting Minnesota. When asked whether he was surprised by the early findings of the Seven Countries Study, Dr. Keys answered, "The big surprise was that what people eat matters. Specifically, that fat in the diet can raise cholesterol in the blood, and in turn can increase heart disease risk. The other scientists didn't believe it...The other surprise, of course, was that different kinds of fat have different effects on serum cholesterol."

Question: "But Americans seem to be getting fatter year by

3. Personal communication with Dr. Henry Blackburn, August 2014.
4. Kromhout D, Menotti A, Blackburn H (Eds). *The Seven Countries Study: A scientific adventure in cardiovascular disease epidemiology.* Brouwer Offset b.v., Utrecht, ISBN 90-6960-048-x, 1994. 219 pp. This monograph can be found in full on the Seven Countries Website: http://sevencountriesstudy.com/study-findings/publications
5. Jaret P. (1997) The man behind the Mediterranean. *Eating Well*, March/April issue, pp. 40-49. www.eatingwell.com

year, according to the latest numbers. Does that worry you?" Dr. Keys answered, "It's something we see every time we come back to Minnesota to visit family. You just don't see so many fat people in Italy as you do in the U.S."

Question: "When you look back at the places you've worked, are you encouraged by what you see? Are people eating better?" Dr. Keys answered, "In some parts of the world, the news is very, very good. Let me give you my favorite example. I've done a lot of my work in Finland, which had more coronary heart disease than anywhere else in the world—and a diet exceptionally high in saturated fat." .... "The last time I was there, four years ago, the Minister of Health met with me and thanks me for saving 2,000 lives a year in Finland. That's the difference between the number of people dying of coronary artery disease before we went in to do our studies–before we convinced them to change their diets—and now."

Question: "When you look back over your career, what gives you the greatest satisfaction?" Dr. Keys answered, "The fact that our findings have held up so well. We were really the first to introduce the whole business of studying populations rather than individuals."... "But what we discovered about fat and cholesterol and heart disease has remained unchallenged. I'm very proud of that."

In 2004 the University of Minnesota launched the First Ancel Keys International Symposium of Nutrition and Health in honor of the long research career of Dr. Keys. The topic of the first symposium was "*The International Obesity Epidemic*." At the symposium, the President of Italy, through a special envoy, gave Dr. Keys the Silver Medal of Merit for his pioneering studies on the Mediterranean diet.[6]

6. Archives of Dr. Ancel Keys and Margaret Keys, and the Seven Countries Study. University of Minnesota Division of Epidemiology and Community Health. Courtesy of Dr. Henry Blackburn. http://www.epi.umn.edu/cvdepi/

Genius

The question that comes to my mind is whether Dr. Ancel Keys was a true genius? After writing most of this book, I can state without doubt, and I will defend my case to the very end, that Dr. Keys was a genius. Why? Dr. Keys spent his entire adult life (see Time Line) learning and searching for answers to important scientific questions. Ancel Keys sought out several major, world-renown scientists, including a Nobel Prize recipient, to work with during his post-graduate studies. After performing studies on human adaptation to extreme stress at very high altitude, he established his own research program at the University of Minnesota in 1939. Granted–this was a special time in American history. After all, one could say that Dr. Keys was a great scientist, but that he was also shaped by the times he lived in–especially during World War II. Many Americans, including millions of American service men and women, were brought forward from their local communities and accomplished amazing achievements during the war. This was best depicted in the story of the "Monuments Men," who in most cases were trained artists or museum technicians, and as soldiers in World War II, performed many acts of courage and heroism in order to save the arts works of European countries (and with them a large portion of their past record of European civilization) from destruction.[7] But Dr. Keys used his knowledge to make exceptional scientific contributions to the war effort.

The reason why the War Department asked Dr. Keys to formulate a light, compact meal for paratroopers was that he had conducted research on high-altitude physiology. They thought he would better understand metabolism better at high altitude. He worked hard to come up with a nutritious, yet palatable meal,

7. Edsel RM, Witter B.(contributor) (2009) *The Monuments Men: Allied Heroes, Nazi Thieves and the Greatest Treasure Hunt in History.*Publisher: Center Street.

and it was so successful that the Army expanded its use across all their forces. The adage that an army moves and fights on its stomach still applies, and maybe American troops had a slight edge in World War II because Ancel Keys did a good job. Also during World War II, Dr. Keys had the foresight to study starvation in conscientious objectors as he knew this would be valuable knowledge. If you read the excellent book by Todd Tucker on the starvation studies, published in 2006,[8] one finding that stands out is that starved subjects will go to extraordinary lengths, even to the point of stealing garbage, to eat extra food. Insights into the physiology and psychology of starved subjects helped the Army and relief agencies prepare for the treatment of liberated starved prisoners and the semistarved populations they encountered at the end of World War II.

Then, in the late 1940s, Dr. Keys went on to study the diets and lifestyles of men who were in the age range of men who were dropping dead all over the United States due to coronary heart disease. But it was here that Ancel Key's true genius shone through. He assembled an international team of collaborators who would help him pull off an incredibly difficult study. And as he mentioned in *How to Eat Well and Stay Well the Mediterranean Way*, there were literally hundreds whom he needed to thank for their help. The main collaborators were the principal investigators who were listed as coauthors on *Seven Countries*. Considering the time (1950s-1960s) that this study was organized and carried out, before computers, commercial jet planes, and the internet, it is remarkable that the Seven Countries Study worked so well and produced such important data. Dr. Keys's ability to assemble a world-class group of scientists was another, and extremely important, manifestation of his genius.

Then Dr. Keys went one step further: in partnership with his wife, Margaret Keys, the two of them produced three major

8. Tucker T. (2006) *The Great Starvation Experiment - The Heroic Men Who Starved So That Millions Could Live*. Free Press (Simon & Schuster), New York.

cookbooks, with *How to Eat Well and Stay Well the Mediterranean Way* being a landmark effort to spread the knowledge gained from the Seven Countries Study. I feel this was the capstone of their remarkable careers!

Partnership

When reading through the archives of Dr. Keys, one is struck by the observation that Margaret Keys is always somewhere in the picture (literally and figuratively–visit the website developed by Dr. Henry Blackburn and the Division of Epidemiology and Community Health: http://www.epi.umn.edu/cvdepi to see the hundreds of photographs and several videos from their travels). Margaret Keys was certainly there on Dr. Keys's first visit to Naples in 1952, where a small study measuring serum cholesterol concentrations was undertaken. Margaret traveled with Ancel during most of the pre-Seven Countries Study period. The photos below show Margaret Keys during the pre-survey of Crete in 1957.

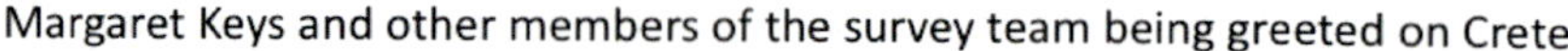

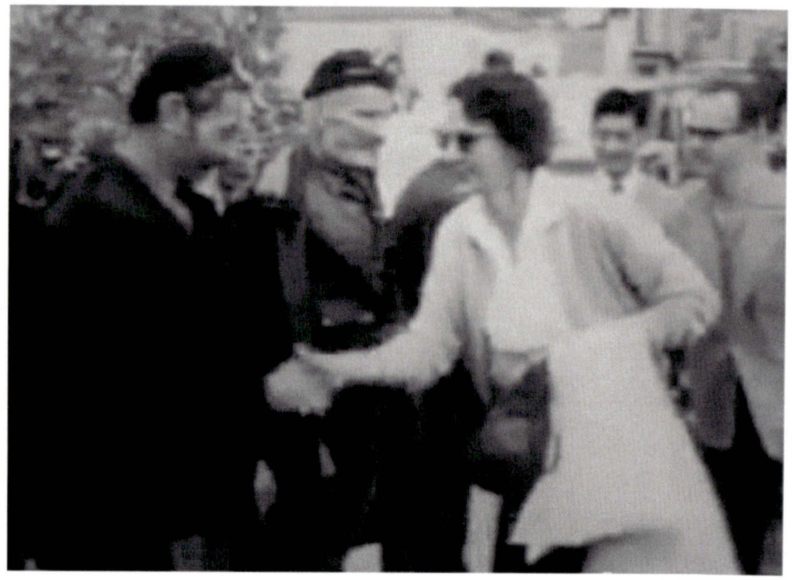

Screen shot from film made of the Crete Pilot Survey during the 1957 pre-studies for the Seven Countries Study. "Italy and Crete Pilot Survey 1957." Video can be seen at: http://www.epi.umn.edu/cvdepi/video/italy-and-crete-pilot-survey-1957/

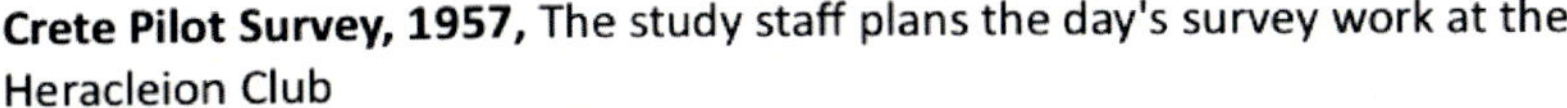
Crete Pilot Survey, 1957, The study staff plans the day's survey work at the Heracleion Club

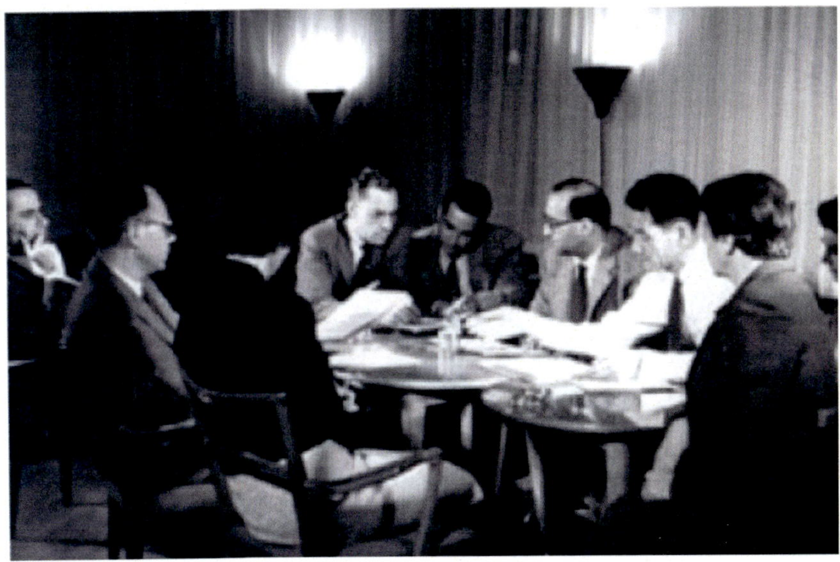

Photo from the Crete Pilot Survey during the 1957 pre-studies for the Seven Countries Study. Courtesy of Dr. Henry Blackburn. Original photo provided by Flaminio Fidanza. See hundreds of photographs at: http://www.epi.umn.edu/cvdepi/multimedia/photographs/

In the first figure, Margaret Keys is being greeted by officials on the Island of Crete. Dr. Keys is right behind Margaret and Drs. Noboru Kimura and Flaminio Fidanzais are in the background.

In the second figure, the study staff plans the day's survey work at the Heracleion Club: from left around the table, Margaret Keys, Alexander Dontas, Christ Aravanis, Ancel Keys, Christ Chlouverakis, Flaminio Fidanza, Noboru Kimura, Cybele Chlouverakis, and an unidentified woman.

In fact, on one particular trip, Margaret Keys may have participated directly in a landmark scientific finding. The picture that was posted in chapter 6 of this book showed Margaret Keys working in the lab during the visit to South Africa. Again I quote from William Hoffman's article in the University of Minnesota's *Update*, Winter 1979: "In 1955 Keys and his wife, Margaret, a biochemist, went to South Africa to begin systematic work on the Bantus, Cape Coloreds, and Europeans. 'She did all the fieldwork,' Keys said.[9] The highly publicized findings showed that the calorie intake of fat varied widely in the diets of the three groups, and blood cholesterol counts and the incidence of heart disease correlated with diet — lowest for Bantus and highest for Europeans."

When I read the original article in the *Lancet*,[10] I was stunned by the findings. This study is interesting and both scientifically and historically important for several reasons. Dr. Keys wished to work with Dr. Brock, a physician in South Africa. The first reason this study is interesting is that it showed how Ancel and Margaret Keys participated together in some of the early pre-studies. Margaret was a laboratory technician/biochemist, who set up the lab and then broke it down everywhere they traveled. I was able to find Margaret's diary entries for this particular period.[11] Below is an abbreviated listing of these entries:

March 6 Arrive Cape Town
March 7 Cape Town Lab all day
March 8 Lab
March 9 Lab 8:30 to 7:30
March 14 Lab
March 30 Leave Cape Town

9. Hoffman, W. (1979) "Meet Monsieur Cholesterol" (Profile of world renowned cardiovascular epidemiologist Ancel Keys). *Update* (University of Minnesota). http://mbbnet.umn.edu/hoff/hoff_ak.html
10. Bronte-Stewart B, Keys A, Brock JF, with the collaboration of Moodie AD, Keys MH, Antonis A. (1955) Serum-Cholesterol, Diet, and Coronary Heart-Disease, An Inter-racial Survey in the Cape Peninsula. *Lancet* Nov 26 1955, 1103-1108 http://www.ncbi.nlm.nih.gov/pubmed/?term=13272336
11. Keys, Margaret. Personal Diary. Archives of Dr. Ancel Keys and Margaret Keys, and the Seven Countries Study. University of Minnesota Division of Epidemiology and Community Health. Courtesy of Dr. H Blackburn. http://www.epi.umn.edu/cvdepi/

The entries show that Margaret Keys worked long hours in the laboratory during the visit to South Africa. Other diary entries show that she worked hard during the various travels associated with the pre-studies. In the South Africa study there were three groups of participants. There were two groups that had relatively low dietary intakes of fat. The Black South Africans (Bantu) consumed about 15% of their Kcal as fat. The Keyses could not find a single case of coronary heart disease among the Bantu. The Cape Coloured people were descendants of those who migrated to South Africa from Asia, primarily from India, Pakistan, and Malaysia, and they consumed an intermediate level of fat in their diets. The group of White South Africans consumed a diet that contained a much greater saturated-fat content, and their blood cholesterol levels were very much higher compared to the other two groups. The second interesting aspect of this study was that the increase in cholesterol detected in the White South Africans occurred in the "beta fraction," which is what we now call the LDL fraction. Margaret Keys actually used paper electrophoresis to separate the blood lipoprotein fractions. This may have been one of the first studies, if not the first, that showed that when the total blood cholesterol increases in a population in response to a diet high in saturated fat, the increase in cholesterol concentration is observed in the LDL fraction. The above study in South Africa was also discussed in *How to Eat Well and Stay Well the Mediterranean Way.*[12]

In March of 2007, Dr. Henry Blackburn gave an eulogy of Ancel and Margaret Keys.[13] The most cogent memories from Dr.

12. Keys A, Keys M. (1975) *How to Eat Well and Stay Well the Mediterranean Way.* Garden City, New York: Doubleday & Company. page 6.
13. Blackburn, Henry. (2007) Ancel and Margaret Keys Remembered. Personal communication from Dr. Henry Blackburn, M.D. Mayo Professor Emeritus, University of Minnesota Division of Epidemiology and Community Health, School of Public Health, 1300 S. Second St. WBOB Suite 300, Minneapolis, MN 55454, November 24, 2014. (See full Remembrance in the Appendix)

Blackburn's many years of interactions and travels with Ancel and Margaret are:

> They were truly both a family and a professional team. Margaret contributed to the earliest scientific pursuits formulating the K-ration. She shopped to get the ingredients for the successive versions of that famous survival ration. ... Their trek to Naples in winter 1952 began the great study of lifestyle and heart attacks that became the Seven Countries Study. Margaret set up the survey laboratory and did the chemistries in that first exploration to compare the eating patterns and cholesterol levels among different cultures. Much of what we understand about individual and cultural differences in risk of heart attack began with that simple comparison. The workers with Mediterranean eating styles had low cholesterol levels and no coronaries. The bankers ate like Minnesotans and had similar high cholesterol and rates of heart attacks. ...
>
> Margaret was equally essential to the Keyses' activity after the Seven Countries Study became more routine than romantic. Their great joint contribution to good health and dining pleasure was their 1959 book, "Eat Well and Stay Well." Ancel wrote the scientific narrative swiftly, eloquently, and clearly. His writing flowed like Mozart's composing, emerging whole, in a single piece, with great clarity and structure of the ideas. But we know who best knew the ingredients and composed the recipes and tested them again and again until they were finally easy—and perfect. The Keys cookbooks were truly a major joint effort. They became best-sellers and now are collectors' items. ...
>
> Ancel Keys wrote his magnum opus on coronary disease in the Seven Countries Study at age 75. In photographs, one sees Margaret citing the data, dictating the references, gathering the material for entry into the narrative and the graphics of that lasting monograph. Together they did everything but the printing. Then she would slip off into the kitchen and lay out the wonders that kept them nourished, healthy, and vital.

After reading these remembrances, I can't wait for the detailed investigation of the lives of Ancel and Margaret Keys that will soon be published by Dr. Sarah Tracy, a distinguished Professor and Historian of Science and Technology at The University of Oklahoma, Norman, OK 73019.

The Importance of Partnerships in Productive Endeavors

There are social scientists who study partnerships and who posit that a successful partnership results in some of the most successful and productive endeavors.

In the June 2009 issue of *The Atlantic* magazine, author Joshua Wolf Shenk wrote about the Harvard psychological adaptation study that has been following 268 men who entered Harvard University in the late 1930s and is still going on today.[14] President John F. Kennedy was a participant, and Ben Bradlee, who was editor of the *Washington Post* for many years and who died in late 2014, was also enrolled in this study. This longitudinal study has been examining very closely the lives of these men for the last 70+ years. The results of the study are complex, but one of the most stunning findings was that an important component found in most happy and productive lives was having a real, close, working partnership–it didn't seem to matter who the partnership was with, just as long as there was a partnership of some kind.

And, of course, Ancel and Margaret were part of a family and raised three children together. This part of their story will be written about in detail in Dr. Sarah Tracy's official biography of Ancel and Margaret Keys, which should be published in the next year. Therefore, Ancel and Margaret had a successful partnership in their worldwide search for the cause of coronary heart disease, and they had a successful partnership at home, too.

Ancel and Margaret Keys had three children, a boy and two girls. Dr. Keys was forced to retire from the University of Minnesota in 1972. He continued working for another 25 years

14. Shenk JW. (2009) What makes us happy? *The Altantic* June 1. http://www.theatlantic.com/magazine/archive/2009/06/what-makes-us-happy/307439/

or so, mostly at his home south of Naples, on the Mediterranean coast. Margaret Keys was at his side during all of this time. Due to many factors (genetics, personal traits, diet) that can't possibly be known for any particular individual, but one would like to think the Mediterranean diet played an important role, Ancel Keys lived to be 100 years old. He died in Minneapolis on November 20, 2004, two months short of his 101st birthday. Margaret died in 2006 at the age of 97. It is safe to say that Ancel and Margaret had a long and productive partnership, and that they were giants in the fields of nutrition and medicine.

Dr. Ancel Keys was a scientist who traveled the world to make important scientific discoveries. In fact, Ancel Keys probably contributed as much to improve American health as any of the other giants in the nutrition field. Because of Ancel Keys, many of us have had our fathers live 20-to-30 years longer than they might have. For this we should be grateful to him, his spouse, Margaret, and the many scientists who collaborated with him on finding the causes of coronary heart disease.

Throughout this book I have discussed Dr. Keys's major accomplishments. The only problem concerning the accomplishments of Ancel Keys is that many of us did not take his advice–mainly because we did not know about his advice. There is no doubt in my mind that Dr. Keys made great advances in science, medicine, and nutrition that greatly improved the lives of most Americans. And there is no doubt that Margaret Keys was a valuable and essential member of the partnership endeavor that led to many of their contributions to science and health. For multiple scientific discoveries, for contributions to the war effort during World War II, for very long and hard travels throughout the world to track down the cause of coronary heart disease, for writing expert, practical, and down-to-earth cookbooks, and for their overall efforts to improve the health and lives of Americans, Ancel and Margaret Keys deserve to be awarded the Presidential

Medal of Freedom. Unfortunately, it will need to be presented to them posthumously.

APPENDIX

Personal Remembrances of Ancel and Margaret Keys by Dr. Henry Blackburn, MD, given March 22, 2007.

Ancel and Margaret Keys Remembered.[1]

Margaret and Ancel Keys were just back from a field trip to Sardinia in 1955 when we first met in the family music room of Minneapolis friends.

Meeting Ancel was a challenge, almost a joust. He wanted to know what you knew and whether, in fact, you knew anything at all. Margaret on the other hand, wanted to know what you were about and what you and your family were doing. Margaret was concerned with comforting the afflicted. Ancel leaned more toward afflicting the comfortable.

They were truly both a family and a professional team. Margaret contributed to the earliest scientific pursuits

1. Blackburn, Henry. (2007) Ancel and Margaret Keys Remembered. Personal communication from Dr. Henry Blackburn, M.D. Mayo Professor Emeritus, University of Minnesota Division of Epidemiology and Community Health, School of Public Health, 1300 S. Second St. WBOB Suite 300, Minneapolis, MN 55454, November 24, 2014.

formulating the K-ration. She shopped to get the ingredients for the successive versions of that famous survival ration.

Her essential role in the grand adventures leading up to the Seven Countries Study is well documented in photographs and in her journal. She set up the laboratory and did the serum cholesterol determinations on their first population survey in the fogs of Slough, near Oxford in fall 1951.

Many have heard about how Ancel during their Oxford Sabattical followed up on the claim by Professor Gino Bergami that heart attacks were rare in the workers of Naples. Ancel, chafing under an intense lecture series in the damp cold of Oxford, decided that such a clue should be run down. Their trek to Naples in winter 1952 began the great study of lifestyle and heart attacks that became the Seven Countries Study.

Margaret set up the survey laboratory and did the chemistries in that first exploration to compare the eating patterns and cholesterol levels among different cultures. Much of what we understand about individual and cultural differences in risk of heart attack began with that simple comparison. The workers with Mediterranean eating styles had low cholesterol levels and no coronaries. The bankers ate like Minnesotans and had similar high cholesterol and rates of heart attacks.

Ancel and Margaret and colleagues went on to South Africa to make comparisons among the European colonials compared to the Bantu and the Cape Colored ethnic groups, finding further confirmation of Ancel's early ideas about diet, lipids, and heart disease.

Margaret was also central to the 1956 expedition to Japan. It was designed to hold genetic factors constant by comparing Japanese across social classes in Japan, and then across cultures: mainland Japanese versus Japanese who had migrated to Honolulu or on to Los Angeles. This pioneering study confirmed the centrality of eating patterns in determining average blood cholesterol levels and eventual risk of heart attack on the scale of whole populations. That became the Keyses' central contribution to knowledge and to preventive practice and policy. These Medical Marco Polos brought home ideas to test more stringently about the sociocultural causes and prevention of heart attack and stroke.

Margaret was equally essential to the Keyses' activity after the Seven Countries Study became more routine than romantic. Their great joint contribution to good health and dining pleasure was their 1959 book, "Eat Well and Stay Well." Ancel wrote the scientific narrative swiftly, eloquently, and clearly. His writing flowed like Mozart's composing, emerging whole, in a single piece, with great clarity and structure of the ideas.

But we know who best knew the ingredients and composed the recipes and tested them again and again until they were finally easy—and perfect. The Keys cookbooks were truly a major joint effort. They became best-sellers and now are collectors' items.

Then came the fruitful joint activity of Margaret and Ancel in planning, building, and embroidering upon their Villa Minnelea. There is scarcely imaginable a more welcoming Shangri-La of good science and good living than their prominence above the Tyrranean Sea.

Dozens of conferences in their grand seminary of pioneers and original thought gave direction to researches around the world in a fellowship of common concern for health. It would be hard to identify in the annals of medicine a more unifying setting than Minnelea.

Ancel Keys wrote his magnum opus on coronary disease in the Seven Countries Study at age 75. In photographs, one sees Margaret citing the data, dictating the references, gathering the material for entry into the narrative and the graphics of that lasting monograph. Together they did everything but the printing. Then she would slip off into the kitchen and lay out the wonders that kept them nourished, healthy, and vital.

Few know the whole of Margaret's strength and contribution to the years of Ancel's decline: her constant awareness, her efforts to help his struggles with reading, computation, and writing, her handling the frustrations of unaccustomed impairments to the formidable productive force that was, for so long, Ancel Keys's. He died a few weeks short of his 101st birthday!

Today, Margaret and Ancel's character and values live on vividly in their family and colleagues and in those who cared so devotedly for them at the ends of their lives.

Henry Blackburn, 22 March 2007

GLOSSARY

Glossary of the most used terms.

Ancel Keys — Professor of Physiology at the University of Minnesota; Started and Led the Seven Countries Study. Subject of this book. Please see the Time Line of his life.

Atherogenic — An adjective used to describe something (a food, a habit, an endogenous substance such as a cytokine) that will increase the development of atherosclerosis.

Atherosclerosis — The complex process of developing plaques or eruptions of the artery wall that begin to impede the flow of blood through the artery. In addition, there can deposits of materials (including calcium) in the artery wall so that it hardens and loses its elasticity.

Blackburn, Henry — A medical doctor who first interned in the University of Minnesota's Laboratory of Physiological Hygiene in 1953 and then joined the faculty of the University of Minnesota where he worked closely with Dr. Keys from 1956 to 1972, and thereafter when Dr. Keys was in retirement. His expertise was in electrocardiography and medical epidemiology, and he traveled widely providing this expertise during the Seven Countries Study. After Dr. Keys retired, Dr. Blackburn was appointed director of the Laboratory of Physiological Hygiene in 1972. In 1979 he was one of the three scientists who became co-directors of the Seven Countries Study. He retired from the University of Minnesota in

1996, but even today (fall 2014), he continues to collaborate on the Seven Countries Study.

Calories — The nutrition calorie is, in fact, the kilocalorie (Kcal). The average intake in women is about about 2200 Kcal per day, and the average intake in men is about 2800 Kcal per day. Throughout the book the abbreviation Kcal is used. However, when I do use the full name calorie, I am referring to the Kcal. For those who study chemistry, the chemistry calorie is the one that can raise the temperature of 1 cubic centimeter of water one degree centigrade. Consuming 2000 chemistry calories would be equivalent to consuming 2 Kcal – this would not get you very far!

Cholesterol — A molecule that is in the lipid family. Cholesterol is a hydrophobic, waxy molecule that contains 27 carbons and four rings that form the classic sterol structure. Cholesterol has a rigid, planer structure and when inserted into a membrane, it makes the membrane stronger and stiffer. Cholesterol is also the starting molecule for the synthesis of steroid hormones. In blood, cholesterol is carried within lipoproteins.

Cholesterol concentration in blood — The amount of cholesterol in blood is measured by an assay that measures total cholesterol (both free and ester forms) in either plasma or serum (the liquid portions of blood). The unit for cholesterol in blood in the United States, and the term used most often in the text, is mg cholesterol per deciliter of plasma or serum (mg/dL). Also, I often drop the mg/dL and just write the basic cholesterol number. A deciliter is 1/10 of a liter. In Europe, the unit for cholesterol in blood is mmol/liter (mmol/L). Conversions: 1 mmol/L= 38.6 mg/dL; 2 mmol/L= 77.2 mg/dL; 3 mmol/L= 115.8 mg/dL; 4 mmol/L= 154.4 mg/dL; 5 mmol/L= 193.1 mg/dL; 6 mmol/L= 231.7 mg/dL.

Coronary Heart Disease (CHD) – This is the term used throughout the Seven Countries Study for diseases of the major arteries of the heart. In some of the papers the term used is coronary artery disease (CAD). These are the same disease and refer to effects observed when the major conduit arteries of the heart are partially to fully blocked, limiting blood flow to heart muscle cells, called cardiomyocytes.

Cohort — This is an epidemiological term that refers to a particular group of people who will be followed together in the study through time. In the Seven Countries Study, men recruited within a certain defined geographical area of a participating country were called a cohort. If different regions were studied within a country, each region constituted a distinct cohort.

Docosahexaenoic acid (DHA) — A 22-carbon fatty acid that contains 6 double bonds. It is one of the omega-3 fatty acids, each of which forms a complex, crooked-shaped molecule. DHA is found in marine organisms because it is mainly synthesized in algae. Therefore, it is one of the fatty acids found in fish oils.

Eicosapentaenoic acid (EPA) — A 20-carbon fatty acid that contains 5 double bonds. Each of the omega-3 fatty acids forms a complex, crooked-shaped molecule. EPA is found in marine organisms because it is mainly synthesized in algae. Therefore, it is one of the fatty acids found in fish oils.

Fat — Fat is the general term for triacylglycerol (abbreviated TAG), the molecule that is made up by attaching three fatty acids to a glycerol molecule. This substance is fairly nontoxic and can be easily stored as a lipid droplet in cells. Triglyceride is another term used for triacylglycerol. Fat is one component in the diverse lipid category. Other major lipids include steroids (cholesterol), phospholipids, and sphingolipids. However, there are over 10,000 different lipids in a cell, including complex lipids of every kind. In the diet, 95% of the lipid in a meal is made up of fat (triacylglycerol). Liquid vegetable oils are nearly 100% triacylglycerol. Fat is stored in adipose cells (also called fat cells), which are specialized cells that are packed full of lipid droplets.

Fatty acid — These long chains of carbon can be found in low concentration (amount) in the body as free fatty acids. Fatty acids (in groups of three) in the body are more often attached to a glycerol molecule to form a triacylglycerol (TAG), which is also called fat. Fatty acids have two ends, the carboxylic acid (-COOH) end, and the methyl (-CH3) end (also called the omega end), located at the end of the "fatty tail."

Heart Attack — When blood flow is impaired in the major conduit arteries of the heart, and the muscle begins to die due to a lack of oxygen.

High Density Lipoprotein (HDL) — A lipid and protein particle that carries cholesterol through aqueous blood. The structural protein of HDL is apolipoprotein A-I. The main job of HDL is to return excess cholesterol from peripheral tissues (including the arteries) to the liver in a process called "reverse cholesterol transport." In most studies, a high HDL concentration in blood has been found to be protective against coronary heart disease.

How to Eat Well and Stay Well the Mediterranean Way — A combination treatise on the Mediterranean diet and a cookbook of recipes, by Ancel and Margaret Keys. The recipes were tested in the Keyses' home. It was published in 1975 by Doubleday, Garden City, NY. In some of the figures in this book, I use the abbreviation: HTEWASWTMW. This cookbook starts off with several chapters that describe how the Seven Countries Study was conceived and implemented.

Hydroxy Methylglutaryl-Coenzyme A Reductase (HMG-CoA reductase) — This is the name of an important enzyme that is early in the synthesis pathway of cholesterol. It is highly regulated: its amount goes up when cholesterol is needed by the cell, and its amount goes down when there is enough or excess cholesterol in the cell. The drug category known as statins inhibit this enzyme so that it cannot work, and thus, statins decrease the synthesis of cholesterol in the cell. When the liver cell senses that it needs more cholesterol after statin treatment, the liver cell increases the number of LDL receptors on its surface membranes, and more LDL is taken up into the liver cell. This has the positive effect of decreasing the amount of LDL cholesterol in the blood.

Intermediate Density Lipoprotein (IDL) — A lipid and protein particle in the blood that is midway between conversion of VLDL to LDL. The protein that surrounds IDL like a belt is apolipoprotein B. The IDL particle carries both triacylglycerol and cholesterol in the bloodstream. In the 1950s John Gofman at the University of California-Berkely published a series of articles indicating that high IDL concentrations in the blood were associated with coronary heart disease. This hypothesis is still being debated by lipid scientists.

Ketosis — The condition that occurs in starvation, or when consuming a very low carbohydrate diet, when fat oxidation increases to provide energy for the body. In ketosis, liver cells incompletely oxidize fatty acids and produce ketone bodies (ketones), which are released into the blood. The ketone bodies cause the blood to become acidic and small amounts are secreted into the urine. Dr. Keys stated that at most about 100 mg of ketones (an insignificant amount in terms of energy) are released into the urine per day.

Low Density Lipoprotein (LDL) — A lipid and protein particle that carries cholesterol through aqueous blood. The protein that surrounds LDL like a belt is apolipoprotein B. The LDL particle carries most of the cholesterol (about 75%) in the bloodstream. In most studies, a high LDL cholesterol concentration is a potent risk factor for the development of coronary heart disease.

Meta-Analysis — A type of epidemiological review study where the published data from many studies are considered and analyzed together and plotted on the same graph in order to determine whether similar effects are observed by the treatment being investigated across many studies.

Mediterranean diet — The diet referred to in this book is the one described in the book, *How to Eat Well and Stay Well the Mediterranean Way,* by Ancel and Margaret Keys. It is also described in detail in Chapter 14 of this book. It is a diet that largely relies upon whole grains, leaf vegetables, and occasionally, seafood. It is low in meat, butter, and other dairy foods. It relies heavily on olive oil and nuts. Wine is often consumed at family meals. The exact description of the Mediterranean diet can differ among publications and studies. The diet in this book is the one described by the Keyses.

Monounsaturated fatty acid (MUFAs) — This is a fatty acid that has only one double bond in its chain, which causes one kink in the structure of the fatty acid such that it looks like a dogleg hole at a golf course. The most common monounsaturated fatty acid is oleic acid, which contains the double bond after the ninth carbon. Oleic acid is very high in olive oil, and is often high in the Mediterranean diet.

Omega-3 fatty acids (ω-3 fatty acids) — These are a specific category of polyunsaturated fatty acids (PUFAs) that contain a double bond at the third carbon from the end of the carbon chain. There are three major omega-3 fatty acids. α-linolenic acid (ALA) is 18 carbons long and contains 3 double bonds and is found in certain plant oils. Eicosapentaenoic acid (EPA) is 20 carbons long and contains 5 double bonds. Docosahexaenoic acid (DHA) is 22 carbons long and contains 6 double bonds. Each of the omega-3 fatty acids forms a complex, crooked molecule. EPA and DHA are found in marine organisms because they are mainly synthesized in algae.

Phospholipids — These are a family of molecules that have two fatty acids on one side and a charged head group that includes a phosphate linkage on the other side of the molecule. When phospholipids line up side by side with, collectively, all the fatty acids facing one side of a plane, and all the charged head groups facing the other side of the plane, the structure formed is called a membrane.

Polyunsaturated fatty acids (PUFAs) — These are fatty acids that have more than 1 double bond. They are usually long chain (have 16 carbons or greater) and the multiple double bonds cause the fatty acid to have multiple kinks in its structure that gives it a very crooked orientation. Vegetable oils are high polyunsaturated fatty acids.

Saturated fatty acids (SATs) — This is a fatty acid that has no double bonds and thus the fatty acid is straight in structure. Meats and dairy products and a few plants such as coconut and palm have a high percentage of saturated fat. No food contains just one type of fatty acid. Foods that have a very high content of saturated fatty acids tend to be solid at room temperature. The content of saturated fatty acids varies in animals and can be affected by the diet of the animal.

Seven Countries — Book written by Dr. Ancel Keys and colleagues and published in 1980 by Harvard University Press. It covers the 10-year follow-up period of the Seven Countries Study. Full name: Seven Countries. A multivariate analysis of death and coronary heart disease. Cambridge, MA: Harvard University Press, ISBN: 0-674-80237-3, 381 pp.

Seven Countries Study — Epidemiological study investigating the role of diet in the development of coronary heart disease (CHD) in 16 different cohorts of men, 40 to 59 years old, who were recruited in the late 1950s and early 1960s from seven countries. In some of the quotes from other sources in this book the study is abbreviated as "SCS." This study continues today as the 50-year follow-up is being prepared for publication.

Trans fats (trans fatty acids) — This is a fat formed when vegetable oils high in unsaturated fatty acids are processed with hydrogen in order to form saturated bonds that turn the oil into a solid. However, the process goes awry and some of the unsaturated bonds are formed again, but in doing so, the bonds form the trans configuration. These types of fatty acids (trans) are more potent than saturated fat at raising blood LDL concentrations. Trans fats have a double toxic effect because they also lower HDL in the blood. After 1990 the food companies began to remove trans fatty acids from their products.

Transcription — The process whereby the cell causes more of a particular protein to be made in the cell with the information coming from the gene in the DNA. Many proteins in the cell are regulated by how much of the protein is synthesized by the cell when the gene is "turned on."

Triacylglycerol (abbreviated as TAG) — It is also known as triglyceride, and commonly referred to as fat. Over 95% of the fat in the diet is in the form of triacylglycerol molecules, which are made up of three fatty acids attached to a single glycerol molecule. This is a relatively nontoxic way to store fatty acids in the body. Vegetable oils, which are almost 100% pure triglyceride, are highly unsaturated and liquid at room temperature. Beef fat is highly saturated and often solid at room temperature.

Very Low Density Lipoprotein (VLDL) — A lipid and protein particle that carries triacylglycerol (TAG) through aqueous blood. The protein, apolipoprotein B, surrounds VLDL like a belt. The VLDL particle carries most of the triacylglycerol in the bloodstream. It is secreted by the liver and its role is to transport fatty acids (in the form of triacylglycerol) from the liver to muscle and heart, and then back to adipose (fat cells). After transport through the blood, some VLDL particles are converted to Intermediate density lipoprotein (IDL) and then further to Low density lipoprotein (LDL).

Western Diet (also known as the typical American diet today) — This diet is a result of our modern culture. As 50% of meals are eaten outside the home, half of this diet is eaten in restaurants and other venues (convenience stores, etc.). On average, 50% of the calories are provided by carbohydrate, 35% from fat, and 15% from protein. About 15-20% of total Kcal come from simple sugars. The fiber intake is relatively low, and in some areas of the United States, there is negligible intake of omega-3 fatty acids.

ACKNOWLEDGMENTS

I would like to thank Dr. Henry Blackburn for meeting me at the Division of Epidemiology at the University of Minnesota and answering a long list of questions about Dr. Ancel Keys. Dr. Blackburn read several versions of the book and sent me difficult to find early articles by Dr. Keys and his group. He also provided the photographs of Ancel and Margaret Keys. Thanks go to Dr. Kenneth Katta for reading a very early version of the book and for sending me a comprehensive set of comments and suggestions. I would also like to thank Mary Steever of Metuchen, NJ, for reading several early versions of the book. Dr. Charlotte Markey of Rutgers Camden was helpful with discussions concerning nutrition and diets and provided many insights into the writing process. Thanks go to Marlene Perchinske for preparing wonderful "Mediterranean" meals in our home on a regular basis. Peter Serko designed the cover and photographed the cover image. My colleagues in the Department of Nutritional Sciences at Rutgers University were very helpful in providing feedback and support for the project. These include Dr. Joshua Miller, Dr. Malcolm Watford, and Dr. Judith Storch. I would like to thank the many students that have taken my Nutrition and Health course over more than 20 years and who inspired me with all their questions and insights. Sincere appreciation goes to Janice T. Pilch, Copyright and Licensing Librarian at Rutgers University, who provided cogent advice on all aspects of the permissions process. And finally, I would like to thank Karen Imperiale, who as my copy editor, made the book look polished and glowing. This book is dedicated to my parents, Leonard and Margaret Dixon, who provided a strong foundation through their unconditional love. The book is also dedicated to Dr. Roger Strair and Advanced Practice Nurse Kara Saggiomo, who tenaciously fought my cancer and allowed me to continue on my journey.

ABOUT THE AUTHOR

Joseph L. Dixon grew up in Brooklyn, NY, and attended Brooklyn Prep High School and later SUNY-Binghamton. He received M.S. and Ph.D. degrees from the University of Wisconsin-Madison. In 1989, he went to Columbia University to study lipoproteins. In 2004, he moved to Rutgers University, New Jersey, which has a strong lipid research group. Dr. Dixon is a lipid biochemist, cell biologist, and an Associate Professor of Nutrition in the Department of Nutritional Sciences at Rutgers University, New Brunswick. He has been teaching courses on Nutrition, including a course entitled, Nutrition and Health, for over 25 years. His specific research interests are lipid metabolism and the mass spectrometry of lipids. His other books can be viewed on his website, http://www.josephldixon.com

73929164R00144

Made in the USA
Middletown, DE
18 May 2018